LOVING LARGE

Patti M. Hall

LOVING LARGE

A Mother's Rare Disease Memoir

DUNDURN
TORONTO

Publisher: Scott Fraser | Acquiring editor: Rachel Spence | Editor: Paula Chiarcos
Cover designer: Courtney Horner
Cover image: istock.com/123ArtistImages
Printer: Marquis Book Printing Inc.

Library and Archives Canada Cataloguing in Publication

Title: Loving large : a mother's rare disease memoir / Patti M. Hall.
Names: Hall, Patti M., 1966- author.
Identifiers: Canadiana (print) 20200164198 | Canadiana (ebook) 20200164236 | ISBN 9781459746367 (softcover) | ISBN 9781459746374 (PDF) | ISBN 9781459746381 (EPUB)
Subjects: LCSH: Hall, Patti M., 1966- | LCSH: Mothers—Canada—Biography. | LCSH: Mothers and sons—Canada—Biography. | LCSH: Brain—Tumors—Patients—Canada—Biography. | LCSH: Tumors in adolescence—Patients—Canada—Biography. | LCGFT: Autobiographies.
Classification: LCC RC280.B7 H35 2020 | DDC 362.19699/4810092—dc23

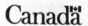
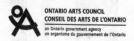
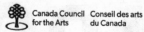
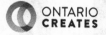

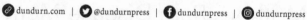

We acknowledge the support of the Canada Council for the Arts and the Ontario Arts Council for our publishing program. We also acknowledge the financial support of the Government of Ontario, through the Ontario Book Publishing Tax Credit and Ontario Creates, and the Government of Canada.

Care has been taken to trace the ownership of copyright material used in this book. The author and the publisher welcome any information enabling them to rectify any references or credits in subsequent editions.

The publisher is not responsible for websites or their content unless they are owned by the publisher.

Printed and bound in Canada.

VISIT US AT

 dundurn.com | @dundurnpress | dundurnpress | dundurnpress

Dundurn
3 Church Street, Suite 500
Toronto, Ontario, Canada
M5E 1M2

To all the giants in my life,
medical, mythical, and magical.

This memoir is a story of my truth, and mine alone. In some instances, I have changed names of individuals and places in order to maintain anonymity, and I have recreated events, locales, and conversations based on my memory of them, however faulty or diluted.

CONTENTS

PREFACE

BECOMING MORE THAN MOM

I wrote *Loving Large* for the *raremoms* and *warriordads* — parents forced on a harrowing, interminable voyage without a map — like more than thirty to forty million families across North America today. The metaphor of being lost at sea resonated with me. My new normal was fearing that the water around me was filled with unspeakably frightening things, and yet I had to move through it, toward a destination no one would ever choose.

We think we comprehend the boundaries of responsibility when we opt in to parenthood. (We think we know a lot of things when we have our babies.) I believed I was a competent mother by the time my kids were in their teens, but I was pulled into unknown waters by duty, loyalty, and love, sure, but primarily by necessity. Because I couldn't find an answer to the one question that drove me to wade in still deeper: *If not me, then who will save my child?*

This is what parents sign up for in the for-better-or-for-worse scenario called Life With Kids. But I was so far out of my depth that I wondered how I would survive without a map or the ability to read the stars. What did that make me? I looked up the origin of *landlubber*. Was it really, as depictions of pirates portray, just *landlover* mispronounced, its edges rounded by windswept, ruddy seamen, who cared less for diction than for drink? Did it mean landsmen — those who've never been to sea? Was it a jab at someone who really should have stayed on land? Or was it an aptly applied label that centuries of usage had morphed into a stigma, a slag? Admiral W.H. Smyth's 1867 digest, *The Sailor's Word-Book*, defined *landlubber* as a sailor's insult for the masses of people who didn't sail and were also unemployed, but other nautical dictionaries add that a *lubber* is a clumsy person and sometimes a lout, and to an able seaman, unseasoned or inexperienced. This would be fairly applied to a newbie sailor who hasn't yet gained her sea legs, I reckoned. A landlubber could be just a person who tipped and wobbled on vessels that were keeling. I've been that landlubber, was she, am her. I was the sailor, the mother, the woman who found herself adrift. The one who lost her moorings.

Although writing was my profession and my passion, and writing to heal one of my specialties, I had to be spurred to write our story at first, and that prompt came from my son. "We should write a blog or something, to tell other people how to find doctors." So I wrote. Aaron changed his mind, or his experience with the disease changed it for him. He waffled about being involved in the telling or not telling of *his* story, ultimately preferring his privacy over reliving the events. But he always supported me writing about it.

As a writing coach, I knew the sound of writer's angst well, but was surprised to hear it coming out of me. I couldn't remember the exhausting anguish of inching forward. What I needed to nudge me arrived in the form of an email from the other side of the world, from a mom whose daughter had a diagnosis and little else. I saw myself in another plaintive, competent, frantic mother, who I thank for this published outcome. Aaron had presented with sore knees. Claire, Toni's daughter, had taut, unbending legs, her ligaments stretched by bones reaching for height her softer tissues were not designed for. My story gave Toni the knowledge that she could endure and her child would survive. Toni was magnificent. She is a medical superhero for Claire. I wrote as if Toni would be my reader.

Loving Large may be *my* book, but it is also *your* story, every parent's story. You don't need to feel alone anymore. We are solo on the voyage, but never alone in feeling lost. Adrift at sea together, we endure because love calls us forward, and so we wade into the dark.

PROLOGUE

VENTURER

I was careful to place my feet between my teenage son's — my feet that were less than half the length of his size fifteens, my painted toenails like ten dropped rose petals on the beige tile floor of the shower.

"Let's do this," I told us both as he shivered, holding the towel around himself, and I checked the water temperature. How many times in his life had I dipped my toe in first or waved my bare hand under the faucet marked H before I let it touch his skin?

The warm streams pressed down on his hair, so thick that it took quite a while to get soaked against the shape of his head. He leaned back to let the water hit his face, to savour the rinsing away of the dingy feeling of being unbathed for so long, of tubes and medical tape and fluids.

We'll be okay. The worst is behind us. Then I noticed the three inches of bloody water around our ankles. And I called my inner voice a fool.

Two months earlier, I was on my phone in my favourite writing spot in a bookstore, where four green leather wingbacks clustered near a fake fireplace. I think what I heard was the doctor asking how he could help. Maybe he said he got my message or he'd heard about my son from whoever found it first. It was his caring tone that cracked me open. Before, I would have mustered a giggle-worthy comeback to make him comfortable, some sarcastic quip to break the tension between strangers, but the last vestiges of my Funny Girl veneer were gone. I'd dismissed her from my cast of characters back in the pediatrician's office. The part of me that could react to crisis went over the cliff's edge as I stared at a pile of my son's school pictures and wondered how the hell I'd missed the signs. By the time the doctor asked the next question, I was managing only mumbles to convey I didn't know how he could help, but I sure as hell needed it.

"Tell me what you know so far," Dr. Graham said.

I blurted out a list of the medical facts I'd gleaned up to that point from doctors with specialties I would previously (and contentedly) not have known existed. Then I rhymed off blood levels and tumour measurements, and when I got to the part about my son's pain, I stood and paced because I thought movement might quell the tears that were rising. I sat back down, just on the edge of the chair at first, but the tenor of the conversation made me feel wobbly, so I slid to the floor, and a few minutes later, I was on my knees. I dissolved into sobs for the first time since I'd heard the word *gigantism* from my son's pediatrician days before. My tears dropped onto the orange carpet, where the little orbs lost their borders, pooling into one almost-red wet spot.

I'd plunged into the Google-verse on the hunt for someone who was expert enough to get my son conclusively diagnosed and tell me what his treatment options were. There had to be an expert somewhere. I didn't know how many doctors it would take to get the information I needed or how far around the globe I'd need to reach for them. Google found a press release announcing an award to a specialist at a California hospital. I clicked the "more info" link and then the "contact us" button.

The endocrinologist on the phone worked with the celebrated doctor, and somehow, he had heard about me already, less than twelve hours after I put some sentences into the online form at some public relations firm in Berkeley, California. I didn't know enough yet to realize that this meant I had a very sick child.

I would never have been so brazen had it been about my health; I'm not the queue-jumping type. I'm more the wait-my-turn kind, the one who lets the customer with just one item slip ahead to the cashier. Being this unabashed for my kids was still foreign to me. I'd never left a middle-of-the-night harried message on the pediatrician's answering service begging for the first appointment. In fact, I hadn't taken either of my boys to the doctor's office for so much as a fever, infection, or minor wound in years.

"You're doing all the right things," Dr. Graham said. Then, quiet. I wasn't going to get the relief I'd desperately wanted. I'd counted on him to tell me about next steps, but he hadn't dropped the details for a cure or told me that hundreds of other kids before Aaron had followed some treatment plan and were fine. I was still clinging to the hope that somebody somewhere (could it please be him?) might hear our story and tell me that this had all been one big mistake. Instead, I was sobbing, wiping my nose, snuffling like an ice-cream-dropping toddler.

"All the right things? You mean we've done *everything* there is to do?" My breathing quickened again. I needed to know what to do. Someone needed to tell me what to do. *There's still more to do, isn't there?*

"Even doing all the right things, it still may not be enough."

What did he just say? I couldn't have heard him right. *Not enough for what?*

I drew in my breath. Panic choked out any calm I was starting to manage. A thousand fears came rushing in.

"All the right things aren't getting us to an expert, Dr. Graham," I told him. "Not the tumour expert, the disease expert, or the brain surgeon we need. All the right things are just leading to more questions, more tests, more prescriptions."

"You'll need all those doctors and more," he replied. I heard his practised calm. He wasn't going to tell me how to find what Aaron needed. I was on my own.

"It's not like I can just call them up." I had a mental picture of me, uber-polite and bubbly on the phone to some receptionist: "Oh, hi.… Can I make an appointment this afternoon with your world-renowned brain surgeon–boss to check out the golf ball–sized tumour in my son's head? Yes, sure, I can hold." My voice was cracking. I was sobbing again, wiping my nose on my coat sleeve. Pleading tones seeped out of me. "It doesn't work that way. At least not where I live. It takes a long time to be seen here and I don't even know who we need to see."

I'm pretty sure that doctors have no idea how difficult it is for patients to get access to them. Specialists, in particular, are oblivious to the long waits, the mystery of how to move up the queue, and helplessness of seeing a condition deteriorate before getting to the doctor. Even best case, it would take months to get Aaron a first consult. I must have said this out loud.

"Knowing what you've told me … in my estimation …" — he hesitated or stuttered maybe on this point — "Your son doesn't have that kind of time." My mouth fell open. I stared, stopped twiddling the pen between my thumb and forefinger.

No back-pedalling followed. He didn't say, "I haven't examined Aaron of course, so I can't be sure.…" And Dr. Graham certainly had every right to *not* give me an opinion at all. He hadn't even seen a photograph or test result. He was taking my word for it. And he'd called me. My kid really *was* in trouble.

"Fewer than a hundred or maybe two hundred children in the world have this condition," he told me, adding that not many more than that were recorded in the last century. There were eight billion people on the globe. How could anything truly be that rare anymore? What would that percentage even be and out how many decimals? *Why my kid? Why here? Why now?* The doctor wasn't done. "Unfortunately, rare as it is, we *do* understand the progression of the symptoms." His voice had gone flat.

I might have been crouching, could have been in the fetal position under a display table. I saw nothing. I felt pressure in the side of my head, as if my eardrum was struggling to get closer to the phone. I could hear the doctor breathing. Was this difficult for him too? Didn't he do this kind of thing every day? Did he know he was calling to destroy my life? I heard something else, something deeper than sound, larger than noise, rising from a sinister place where dark truths about children hide until frailty and hopelessness allow them to emerge. First a rumbling and then a ticking, uneven and random, settling at last into a rhythm, the cadence of a countdown. *Tick. Tick. Tick.* It had been running down for months, maybe years, before an eagle-eyed technician found my son's tumour on a CT scan.

How much time is left?

I hadn't even had a conversation with my husband about the lengths we might have to go to get Aaron care. Like everyone else who'd passed time in waiting rooms leafing through out-of-date dog-eared copies of *Reader's Digest*, I knew the stories; I'd heard accounts of kids travelling halfway around the world to get to medical experts.

"Do we need to bring my son to California? Are you guys the only place that can treat him?" And then, "Can *anyone* treat him?"

I couldn't fathom the kind of planning that travelling for an unknown amount of time across the country would entail. There was the cost and Aaron's schooling and keeping his little brother's life on an even keel. There was my husband's work, our home, families, and animals. But I had to ask that question, no matter how much I loathed the idea of begging this big-city doctor for help.

How the hell did this become my family's story?

I

HANDLER

About a month before that phone call, before I heard the ticking of the bomb that had been dropped on us, our life was a happy chaos, but not noteworthy by any stretch. It was never easy to get my boys to do anything they didn't want to do, including going to the doctor for regular checkups. I chose my battles with Aaron and Justin deliberately and sparingly. I admired their tenacity and secretly took a little bit of credit for it. We parented them with this priority, that they would feel listened to, something both Rick and I had found lacking in our own childhoods. And somehow together we built our family around the importance of expression.

Once after an uneventful checkup, our pediatrician said, "Patti, don't bring the boys in unless you really think they're sick, because the germs in the office are a greater risk than waiting a little longer." I always felt like I needed a hazmat suit in the place, so I took her advice. And the boys were never sick, so that made it easy to avoid the germ-pit. They were also resilient. I'd been the trainer on their hockey teams, witnessing them playing on after taking pucks in the face and getting elbowed in the kidneys.

On this cold, snowy January day Aaron was protesting that he didn't want to go to school, saying he was in too much pain. Pain? He had my full attention. "Something's really wrong with my knees, Mom. There's no way I can do gym. It hurts too much. And it's friggin' impossible to walk up the fifty flights of stairs in that million-year-old school."

I was listening, but I also knew my kid. Aaron's personality had a tinge of the dramatic. He would play through, but more often than not, his bruises were "agony" and his cuts were "lethal" when I got his teenager-style earful afterward. Justin was the opposite. He once walked around with a gaping leg wound caused by the chain on his bike, content to rave proudly about the distance he'd been thrown in the fall ("You wouldn't believe it, Mom!") while wiping at the blood with his grimy pant leg. But something about Aaron's piteous descriptions told me not to shrug this one off.

So I called the pediatrician's office, even though I felt silly taking him out of school and driving a half hour for a doctor to feel his knees. I was sure I'd be dropping him at school later feeling like a hovering, paranoid mother with too much time on her hands.

I ran through all the possible outcomes on the way there, a project manager by instinct and profession. *Worst case: He has a previously undiagnosed injury or juvenile arthritis. Outcome: He'll need some medication for pain or inflammation, maybe a test. Best case: It's growing pains. Outcome: She'll tell him to push through, ice it, take a little ibuprofen.* Either way, I wanted him to hear it from Dr. Tobin. Aaron wasn't going to keep moving through these sore knees for me. I was only his mother. Overruling me was a source of pride, a veritable rite of passage for a fifteen-year-old guy. I'd be going home embarrassed at pushing the panic button, but my kid would learn about endurance. Life lesson achieved.

Small children, mommies, and the staff behind the reception desk looked up casually at first and then almost in unison when Aaron entered the office. The door frame was an eight-footer, and he didn't need to duck to clear it as he stepped into the Lilliputian space tailored for preschoolers and toddlers. The coat hooks hung at my waist height, about mid-thigh on Aaron, and cushioned benches below my knees rimmed the large open area, skirting a pastel broadloom that mimicked moss-covered rocky outcrops. The other parents, with babes in arms and infants in carriers, couldn't resist ogling my six-foot-five teenager. He took up so much space. I might've stared too.

"What are they lookin' at?" he mumbled, so only I could hear.

"You're hot," I whispered back.

Aaron grinned, towering over me at the reception counter. "That is just plain creepy coming from my mother."

"Suck it up, Buttercup."

"Wow, it's been eight years since you've been in," the receptionist told us. "Our records have been through a flood." She pulled a crinkled dirty-looking manila folder into view and held it like a dead rodent, by the corner. The ink on Aaron's chart was smeared, the outside speckled with mould.

Dr. Cathryn Tobin wore the same casual anti-uniform she'd sported when I met her sixteen years before: black jeans and a crisp white shirt with Disney characters embroidered on the chest and lapels. She was maybe four foot ten, which, combined with her warm smile, friendly disposition, and ability to slip into kidspeak with her patients, made it difficult to guess her age. Her bright-blue eyes crinkled at the edges and closed when she smiled, a trait I would call cute, but never to her face. Grey strands salted her soft dark curls, and I happened to know that she had four children older than mine, putting her around fifty.

We followed her past the white salad-bowl-shaped infant scale, where I'd placed my premature son day after day in the first weeks of his life, as Dr. Tobin had hovered, counting precious ounces. We passed the four-foot-high Dora the Explorer jungle-themed measuring stick that was just over belt height on Aaron (chest height on me) on our way into a tiny mauve examining room that featured a Tinker Bell mural. The point of Tink's teeny gold wand was poised to touch the blood-pressure cuff mounted on the wall. I perched on the parent seat in the corner, a toddler-sized plastic stool. Aaron slouched against the examining table, hands in the pockets of his baggy low-slung jeans. He rested a high-cut Nike sneaker on the tiny blue staircase placed there for little ones to clamber up onto the paper-covered table.

"Hop up," Dr. Tobin said out of habit, and we all chuckled when she looked up from the file to see that the exam bed's top caught him in the back of the thigh. "I guess you won't need the steps, then." She nodded to the little stairs and his big shoe. "How tall are you now, Aaron?"

"I think I'm about six-five." She flipped to the cover sheet on a fresh file and ran her pen down his vital statistics. "You'll be sixteen soon."

"Two weeks," he said.

Had he not been at the centre of it, Aaron would have seen the comedy in all of this. Dr. Tobin had seemed little even when she assisted at his birth, holding all five pounds thirteen ounces of him in her delicate hands. She looked up at Aaron and reached to palpate his thyroid as he sat with legs swinging on the raised exam table — it would have made for a great viral video. But a feeling of seriousness had enveloped our group once the door closed behind us; it wasn't the time to joke with Aaron about how not-kid-like he looked in this space.

Dr. Tobin plotted Aaron's height onto a sheet stapled inside the cover of the chart. "You've always been off the chart for height," she said. Then she pressed the soft tissue around his knees and manually levered each leg up and back to listen for clicks with the stethoscope and without. "It looks like Osgood-Schlatter Disease."

Aaron and I both leaned in and asked, "What?"

"It happens when bones and ligaments grow at a different rate and it has a lot to do with growth plates not closing," she said. "It's an inflammation on the shinbone basically, where the ligament is attached to the patella. Your kneecap."

Instant relief. *It was something simple. Something with a name. Good, I didn't waste the doctor's time bringing him in.*

Dr. Tobin turned to Aaron, resting her hand on his knee and looking him directly in the face. "I think we'll do an X-ray to be sure."

Aaron made a strangled noise. He was stricken, gone pale. "Will it hurt?" he blurted, looking down into his lap. Although there had been some crises in his infancy, other than the required vaccinations and a broken bone in his elbow when he was five, there'd been no medical interventions in years, not so much as a prescription.

"No, it's no big deal," Dr. Tobin reassured him. "You'll sit up on a kind of cold metal table while a technician positions your leg and takes pictures of your bones. It'll take less than five minutes." She could see Aaron's tear-filled eyes, how he fidgeted, lifting each leg in turn to jam his fingers under his thighs, and the dappling of sweaty spots on his red T-shirt. *I didn't know who to be for him in that moment. He was almost sixteen. Would it embarrass him if I hugged him? Would he tell me to get away? I didn't know which was worse. I didn't know whose feelings to protect, Aaron's or my own. I knew I shouldn't care about his reaction, but I also knew that Aaron's pride was the one thing that mattered in that moment. Back off, Mom, I told myself.*

Dr. Tobin returned to her post at the end of the examining table, opened the file again, and held her pen to the top of a blank page. "I just want to ask you some other questions to update the chart."

We had a diagnosis. Weren't we done? I studied the doctor's face instead of asking questions that might reveal my emerging disquiet to Aaron. She was as calm now as she'd been all those years ago, taking him still briny and naked from the obstetrician's hands into the shadowy corner of the birthing suite, just before midnight, where an illuminated incubator kept vigil on the day of his frenzied, frightening early birth.

"Do you have pain anywhere else?" Dr. Tobin asked.

"Just my head," he answered, giggling to himself, expecting her to let it go at that.

She looked at me.

"He's serious," I said, trying not to meet Aaron's eyes, which were burning a hole in my skull.

"Mom, don't! It's no big deal." He was being loud, rude, and he wasn't going to stop.

"He gets a headache almost every day," I said, feeling his glare. I had to tell her. I might not get him here again.

"Mom, not *every* day," he corrected.

"Aaron, when do the headaches happen?" Dr. Tobin asked, breaking the tension.

"At about three o'clock and they get worse with the bouncing on the school bus on the way home. And *not* every day," he added again as a jab for me.

"I send Tylenol to school with him. It usually goes away with one or two extra-strength," I said.

More questions. How long had the headaches been happening? Did they come at other times? Where on his head would he say the pain is? Aaron pointed to the back of his head on the right side just above the ear. Dr. Tobin scribbled more notes. He held his right arm out from his body while she secured the blood-pressure cuff. She took it once, then adjusted the cuff and took it again. "It's higher than I'd like," she stated simply, "but that could just be the anxiety, buddy."

The next question sucked the air out of the room.

"Mom, does Aaron look like his brother?" She was mentally flipping through a diagnostic manual. The onion-skin pages were turning frantically for me too. A month before, my hairdresser, Vicki, had glanced at the boys' school pictures after she'd asked me, "Do they have your curls?" She'd passed the photos back to me and said flatly, "Aaron has acromegaly. You know, gigantism."

"Fuck off!" I'd blurted.

Vicki's mother had acromegaly and was recovering from brain surgery. She had facial disfigurements, her hands were the size of dinner plates, her fingers had outgrown her jewelry, and her shoes had gone up two sizes that year. Poor Vicki. When illness touches your life so closely, you see it everywhere. I was even mildly insulted on Aaron's behalf. I knew acromegaly had a nasty reputation for distorting a person's looks. What did she think she saw in Aaron's picture? He looked like Aaron to me. I loved that face and I'd know if something that serious was wrong with my kid, goddamn it.

But still, that night I'd typed *gigantism* into a search engine. The screen filled with titles and shortcuts, summaries and links. It was overwhelming, not in the way I imagine looking for a needle in a haystack would be, but rather like scanning the surface of the sea waiting for a single breaching whale. I read a long list of symptoms. Sure, if I really thought about it, some of them could apply to Aaron, like sweating a lot, but some absolutely did not. The whole thing was ridiculously unlikely. Vicki was an alarmist. I closed the laptop.

Dr. Tobin's question hung in the air. My husband, Rick, and I had always remarked on how the boys looked so different from one another. We savoured their individuality, even though we loved to remind ourselves of how they resembled each of us too. I think all parents do that. I tried to envision photographs of Aaron and Justin side by side. I'd taken hundreds of them, and I often responded to quizzical remarks about how different my boys looked by saying, "I got one of each — a dark one and a light one." Aaron had thick dark curly hair and Justin's mop was fine and wavy, still very fair, although he wasn't the sunny blond-haired kid he'd been when he started school. Their body shapes were similar, but Aaron was getting fleshy around his middle and across his shoulders. It was time for him to start filling out, I'd surmised. He couldn't stay a skinny kid forever. Then their faces. This was a tender subject for me. My mother had remarked to me many times that "if it wasn't for Justin's curly blond hair" — a very common feature on my side of the family —"you wouldn't know there was any of you in him at all." She always conjoined this with the caveat, "I don't mean he isn't as handsome as Aaron," and she was careful to skirt the edge of the blatant insult, that to her it was a real shame that Justin looked to be entirely a product of Rick's family. A great deal of her favouritism was linked to how my children looked. The fact was, neither Aaron nor Justin looked much like me at all, with their brown and hazel eyes respectively (mine are blue), their darker skin, squarish faces, and thick features. "Doesn't that bother you, Patti? You do all that work getting the boys into the world and they look so much like Rick?" someone would tease. Rick or I would offer back some version of "Wouldn't it be worse if the boys didn't look like their father at all?"

I needed to answer Dr. Tobin's question. Aaron's face was fuller, his chin more pronounced, his nose much broader than his brother's — and much broader than it had been even a year ago. They *had* looked more alike years before, like on our family trip to the West Coast in 2008, I thought with a startle. And Aaron, only two years older than Justin, was eighteen inches taller. I mentally scanned the photos my sister, Kelly, and I had taken of our four children together at the zoo the summer before. We took one every year; it was a tradition. Her daughters, Michelle and Laura, then nine and eleven, were stairsteps below Justin, who had been thirteen. Aaron had stood on the far right, a bronze sculpture of a Komodo dragon behind him, and he was almost twice little Michelle's height.

I crouched on the plastic stool, fighting the compulsion to drop my head into my hands in front of Aaron.

"No," I told the doctor. "They don't look alike." Whatever course she was plotting, we were going there too.

I drove us just a couple of minutes to a local clinic for the knee X-ray, hoping to check off the first item on Dr. Tobin's list.

I pulled in, parked, and chirped my usual, "Let's go, buddy," as I began to get out.

"I'm not going," Aaron said. His arms were folded across his chest.

Leaning back into the car, I said, "It's an X-ray, pal." I closed my door and waited to hear his open. I didn't. Coming around to the passenger side, I pulled up on the door handle; he'd locked it. *This is ridiculous.* I tried my no-big-deal Mom voice through the closed window of the car. "C'mon, Aaron, let's go." I used his formal name, a rarity; he'd been A-man to us since birth.

He was in a rage, growling almost. "You can't make me do this. I know it's going to hurt. I'm not havin' all these tests done. There'll be needles. This is *my* body. Forget it!"

I adopted the attitude of the toddler's mother who, unfazed, walks from the grocery store holding the hand of a screaming two-year-old. I would handle this. I had the key fob in my hand and could unlock the doors, but what was I going to do, yank my huge son by the arm from the car? I could just picture it. Tweety Bird and Sylvester the Cat, unlocking and locking the doors in an endless cycle. So, I stood there while my son threw a tantrum, tears streaming down his angry red face. Over an X-ray. *What the hell am I gonna do when an actual needle is involved?* I waited it out, memories of teary Montessori school drop-offs flashing through my head, how he used to cling to my leg like an octopus until the kindly Mrs. Petrie peeled him from me.

I manifested firm-mom voice. He gave me the stink eye. Then, seventies television show cliché as it was — and I'm *not* proud to admit it — I called his dad and passed my cell through the window crack. Aaron emerged from the car angry as a pit viper five minutes later, handed me my phone, and stomped beside me to the lab door. *At least he didn't smash the phone.*

The X-ray was completed in about two minutes. Aaron hobbled in, hobbled out, and acted like a hero for doing it.

"So, I get ice cream now, right?" he said, grinning at me from the passenger seat.

"You're kiddin' me! After the show you just put on and how you treated me, you think I should be getting you ice cream?" It wasn't an angry tone. I never had one of those. I was so relieved that I couldn't quite dredge up the mock-annoyed tone I was aiming for. He wouldn't have bought it anyway. He knew I was a marshmallow.

"Well, I *was* an awfully good boy, Mom." Playing his half of the comedy duo.

I turned to Aaron and saw the smile ear to ear. We'd survived, intact. I sighed. "You certainly *were*, Big A!" I replied, as though placating a toddler. I should have tousled his hair for good measure. I was glad he'd recovered so quickly, but I was wrung out, as if I'd lived his experience on top of my own.

Aaron dozed while I drove north to our country home, alone with my self-talk. *This will turn out to be nothing. Just a little taste of a scare, enough to spook me, remind me not to take the boys' health for granted. Just get the tests done. And learn this fucking lesson.* Maybe I'd gotten lax and this was my comeuppance. The universe had cuffed me in the jaw, issued a wake-up call, just in case I was getting cocky. I resolved that somehow I had to drag Aaron through the tests, I had to see Dr. Tobin's list through even if he was resistant and belligerent, or I'd always wonder if I should have. We'd be cranky with each other, but after getting cleared for anything seriously wrong, we'd move on and return to the luxury of being unconcerned about health.

Denial: living life in fuzzy slippers, cozied up in a hand-knit blanket from my grandmother, my unrelenting inner voice looping, *It isn't true*. If I didn't look at it, it wasn't there. Like a baby playing peek-a-boo. But somewhere in the background, I could almost hear Elisabeth Kübler-Ross, her accented *r*'s rolling, as she recounted the story of a man who didn't cling to his denial for long because he couldn't afford to. I savoured her work on death and dying. I'd listened to her in many documentary videos while seeking a compelling structure for a book I was writing about a man confronting pancreatic cancer. Her life's work was about so much more than her oft-debated five stages of grief. She got us to talk about how we receive the worst of bad news, about what dying people want, about how diagnoses transform the way people live while they are dying. I had witnessed denial many times as a caregiver; now here I was dabbling in it. *Well, it works for everyone else.*

Aaron was able to move quickly past the anxiety attack over the X-ray; his resilience was alive and well. And he got a shit-ton of bubble gum–flavoured ice cream.

2

MISSION SPECIALIST

Mornings in my house were mitigated bedlam. Aaron and Justin were just coming into the age when sleeping was much preferred to waking up or doing virtually anything else, especially on school days. Calling morning threats into their blanket mounds was standard operating procedure, progressing from plaintive verbal appeals to insistent bellows, with increasing levels of threat. "I'm coming in there." "I'm calling your father." "Do I need to use the water pistol?" As the number of repetitions increased, they were punctuated by pleas for the boys to consider showers, followed by responses to their panicked queries that always began with "Mom, where's my ..." Add to the melee the care and feeding of one cat, one rabbit, and three dogs, one of whom, Reef, was a puppy in training to be a service dog, who needed particular food, daily grooming, and a bag of doggy equipment to be packed for his day.

I pounded grooves in the hardwood floors finding things, letting out, letting in, collecting bowls and glasses, feeding, reminding, and packing. I'm doubtful that chaos theory originated in my kitchen, but I was actively enrolled in a personal program to tame it, every single day. And I was good at it. Inside me, the maelstrom was vicious, but the boys bobbed along in the relative calm of the riverside eddies, because I was on the job.

It was a Monday, Aaron had a CT scan the Friday before and a training day for Reef. That meant three drop-offs. And a few hours later, after I squeezed in groceries, errands, and essentials for the family, it was followed by picking up. One of the boys had band practice in the morning. Both of them had hockey after school. I reminded them of this in the mudroom when they were yanking on coats, then again in the car, and a final time as they got out of the car. It was critical to the dynamic that my boys knew what was coming next. Surprises and their attendant anxiety were to be avoided at all costs. I'm a prevention-style parent, preferring to avoid the explosion than repair the drywall after.

While the boys crammed in cereal, careful to slop as much milk on the counter as possible and never able to quite propel their bowls the whole eighteen inches to the dishwasher, I packed the car, mentally ticking off the essentials with each trip up and down the staircase, through the garage, and outside to the driveway. Loading the car was like provisioning a navy frigate. In went Reef and his bag, a bin of snacks, two backpacks, a traveller cup of coffee, that day's musical instrument, a poster-board homework assignment, gym bags, and permission forms to be handed over the seat at the last moment.

I rushed by the steadily accumulating pile of boxes packed and stacked in the bay of the garage. It was getting more and more difficult not to feel anxious as I stepped around them. One of these mornings the boys were going to notice and ask me what was in those boxes, and that was a conversation I wasn't ready to have. I shook the thought away and focused on the mission at hand. The day going right meant calm for my family, peace for me. And I yearned for peace so badly given the undercurrents of disruption percolating like tiny cauldrons in the boxes I was surreptitiously packing.

The three of us and a gangly-legged golden retriever puppy climbed into our vehicle for our daily foray. I edged the car into the world, fender slipping over the invisible line of the meta-phoric gate I closed each night when we returned home. Now it was heaved open by some imaginary gatekeepers I'd screened a thousand times before giving them the job of keeping my family safe at the Big Blue House in the country.

School drop-offs were at different times in different towns. Aaron was in Grade 10. Justin was still in elementary school. The twenty-minute car ride was an adventure in tossing snacks, which we called our "hobbitses' second breakfastses," into the back seat and featured me interjecting every third sentence to correct someone's language or remind the boys to speak kindly to each other. A phone call from Dr. Tobin's office perforated the seal. The laws hadn't tightened around lifting a cell to your ear while driving, and I answered.

"Dr. Tobin would like you to come in tomorrow at two o'clock," the nurse told me. "And she asks that you not bring Aaron with you."

I glanced in the rear-view mirror and saw that Aaron and Justin were each looking out the window.

"Oh. Okay. I'll be there." *Why is the nurse calling me and not the receptionist?* I returned the phone to the seat beside me, laying it on top of my open daybook, where lists of to-do's and the well-managed timing of everything in our lives lay, like maps on a ship's chart-table.

Dr. Tobin wanted me to come in to the office. Without my kid. *This is about more than letting Aaron skip some track-and-field practice.* She wouldn't need to see either of us in person to discuss that. I supposed that she wanted to talk to me about the CT scan, which we had just days before.

I had experienced the Diagnostic Imaging Department with Aaron years before. Dr. Tobin had sent me with infant Aaron for an emergency CT scan after finding a suspicious pocket of fluid on my newborn baby's scalp. In 1993 I had a fussy baby, along with his stroller, diaper bag, health card, and birth certificate, and no extra hands.

Sixteen years later, the details were still sharp. The extremely wide white door that opened out into the hallway to allow patients to be wheeled through in their hospital beds. The large red-and-yellow warning signs on the wall: Pregnant Women Should Avoid This Area. Radiation Exposure. Both times I'd been there, I supplied the standard response to the parental question, "Yes, I'm the mother." I quickly wrote the same full name, date of birth, and birthplace (that very building), but when I got to "condition presenting with," my hand halted. I glanced over my shoulder. Aaron had left my side and was seated in the chair nearby. When he was a baby, I'd written "cranial scan re fluid on cranium." Now I scrawled "cranial scan — attribution for headaches." I held my cold, damp forehead in my left hand, deliberately avoiding the receptionist's glance as I passed her the form. She likely saw this all the time. The distraught parent sent by the overly cautious pediatrician following up on the wild chance this kid's headaches were more than dehydration. It was likely so routine that she was blasé, annoyed about it even, thinking it was another wasted test. Overzealous mother. Litigation-fearing pediatrician. The receptionist read the form and looked up at me. I felt my chest tighten and realized I was holding my breath.

I hoped the young woman in teddy bear scrubs wouldn't ask a question out loud that might set Aaron off. He hadn't asked what the test might find or what Dr. Tobin was looking for. So far there had been no resistance antics or asshole behaviour, but the X-ray incident was top of mind. If he threw a fit here, at least a hundred people were going to have ringside seats and it was a no-cellphone area, eliminating my last resort, calling Rick. I had no crew on this sortie.

Almost nothing in the place had changed. Seated across from Aaron, who was watching a kid's television show on the screen over my head, I looked around the waiting area. The fear I had felt when he was a baby had both etched some details on my mind and permanently erased others. The yellowish light of the large windowless waiting room, the chairs all facing the televisions, the irritating beeps and repetitive noises of latches closing, and the smells of cleaning solvents, laundry detergent, and Dettol all revisited me. The tan carpeting and the denim-coloured chairs. *Easily sanitized*, I thought. I hated that I could remember this hospital area so perfectly but wasn't able to recall the beautiful details of my sons' faces when they were born.

I'd been a first-time, very cautious mother of a premature baby. "He must lie absolutely still," the CT suite staff told me. *Yeah right*, I'd thought. *He's a newborn. It isn't like I can tell him to be still and he will be.* "Do what you have to," they said, "but keep him still." I watched from inches away as my wailing, wide-eyed baby was placed, limbs spread like a starfish, into a body mould's bottom half. When the top of the mould was pressed down, he looked like a living gingerbread man. I could see only his eyes, nose, and chin. I locked my eyes on his as he kept shrieking. As the table conveyed tiny Aaron back into the belly of the gigantic machine, someone placed heavy leaded blankets over my head and shoulders. ("Is there a chance you could be pregnant, ma'am?" *Do the math!* "Uh, no.") I shook visibly, teeth chattering. At some point the conveyor bed activated and Aaron slid too far inside the machine for me to see his eyes over the height of the mould. His wailing stopped. The sudden silence, which I hoped meant calm, was instead baby Aaron's breath catching in horror at the movement of the table and the change of view. Which he announced moments later with rapid-fire screams filled with the breathlessness of pure fear. My body reacted instantly; my breasts fully engorged. I clambered up onto the table, my shoes dropping to the floor, reaching my open hand deep into the tube to touch him, make skin-on-skin contact with him anywhere.

"You need to get him to calm down or this is useless to us," came through the speaker. I wanted to say, *Listen, you son of a bitch, can't you see that's my baby in there and there might be something wrong with him?* Maybe they missed the empathy unit in college. With my left arm fully outstretched across the hard plastic body mould, I found Aaron's little mouth and offered the knuckle of my index finger. It brought the screaming down to rapid breathing and snuffling. I knew he would reject the knuckle quickly; he'd gotten used to my breast and could not be tricked. With my free fingers I rubbed the silkiness of his chin. I was going to have to start singing soon.

Just days before, in the early throes of postpartum depression, I'd wondered if I'd ever feel that all-consuming, give-up-everything-for-my-baby maternal instinct to care for this little person. I was convinced in the frightening hours after his birth that I was in fact, the worst person to care for him and that I should just let my mother do it. Now I was raging like I was all he had to defend him in this world.

I could never go back to when I just had to worry about myself. It was on me to keep him alive now, well, and happy even, and I'd never felt less capable of anything. Reckoning with the burden of motherhood and my total culpability in that moment must have kept at bay some of the fear of what that scan might find, because I don't recall running scenarios in my mind.

I'd had fewer than three weeks with him, yet I found the song and sang out loud, fully audible to the three technicians peering through the Plexiglas window. I sang Celine Dion's "Water from the Moon," a promise that I would keep trying for him, that I would do anything for him. I'd turn the sand into water. I'd get water from the moon.

Heading down the cold hallway of the hospital with my grown son clomping behind me, the sound of his untied shoe-laces ticking the terrazzo floor, I remembered the previous walk vividly. I felt some solidarity with that sobbing, stressed-out young mom who had assumed the requisite responsibility and savoured the relief of that CT scan showing "nothing sinister." But I was just as alone now. Society tells us it takes a village to raise a child. Where was my village then? Where was it now?

"Hey, A-man, we were here before. When you were a baby," I told Aaron as we took our seats outside CT Scan Room 1. He tried to act interested. Neither one of us could fake it for the other.

"I want this to be over," he said.

I put on my no-big-deal voice. "I know you do. It'll be fast," I said. I told him there would be a machine, that he would lie back on a table, and that although he wouldn't be able to see the technicians, he'd be able to hear their voices.

"You're coming in with me, right?"

"I can't, buddy."

"You did when I was a baby." He was right, damn it all.

"It's really not safe, though, and they won't let me, I'm sure."

"I need you to come."

"It's easier than even the X-ray, and" — I stammered a little, not wanting to use the age card — "you're almost sixteen. You go on in." I hated saying this to him, using his age to shame him. It went against all my intentions for mothering, but I was desperate that he not have a meltdown or simply refuse. *Empower him. I have to get him to do this, somehow. There might be scarier things to do after this.*

Other patients petered away to their own appointments and lives, leaving only Aaron and me waiting. Finally, a tall, thin thirty-something man bounce-stepped the fifty feet or so down the hallway toward us and said, "You must be Aaron, eh? Follow me, buddy." I didn't like him calling my kid *buddy*, but I hoped Aaron would be more at ease with a relaxed guy. "You can stay here, Mom," the tech said to me as he swept his hand in front of him, directing Aaron down the hall. They turned left at the end of the corridor toward another CT suite, leaving me alone in the hallway of chairs. I was relieved to not have strangers around. I'd been alone for so many of the challenging moments in the last twenty years. Rick's work and our decision for me to be home with the children when they were young and later to pursue my writing career from home meant I was the hands-on one tackling most of the tough things with the boys.

I got up to pace, walking with my hands jammed inside my coat pockets, listening to the annoying sound of my boots clicking on the floor, conspicuous in the hushed hospital atmosphere. I hated people with noisy shoes. I started to tiptoe. With no baby to clutch this time, I hugged Aaron's hat and coat to me. *Please, not my baby … please, not my baby …*

Four chairs to the corner, eight on the opposite wall. *Click, click, click.* Two hats, one red and one a polka-dot baby's cap, lay with a hunter-green plaid scarf in a well-handled box someone had cut from the bottom of a Campbell's soup carton, an impromptu lost-and-found. *How long has he been gone? Two lengths of the hall, or has it been three?* I tried perching on the edge of a chair, my arms across my chest, but my eyes filled as soon as I sat down and looked at the floor. *Holy shit, I'm in the hospital getting Aaron a brain scan.* I couldn't let Aaron see me with swollen eyes and a red nose when he came out, so I stood up and took up pacing the floors again, my boot heels keeping time with my breaking heart.

"Mrs. Hall, can you come in and be with your son? He'd like you to come in." The overly enunciating technician had come up the hall behind me. "This is always more difficult than we think it should be." I had no idea what he meant, but I heard his condescension. *Does he think my kid is older just because he's six five? He's just a kid.* Panic had hit me, my hand was on my chest. "It is a brain scan after all," I said, and I was on the move.

I didn't care if the tech thought I was coddling my son or even if he was judging Aaron for being upset; my boy asked for me. I swung into Mom on a Mission. I clicked right into Scan Room 2, where I saw a machine shaped like a massive white donut swallowing Aaron.

"Here's Mom, dude," the tech called to Aaron. There was the hump of him, curled on his side. I dropped everything just inside the door: my bag, coats, iPod, book, and his extra clothes and went to the table. He looked up at me, eyes filled with tears. I glanced at the butterfly needle in his arm and saw what I assumed was the contrast fluid moving slowly into him. He'd been terrified there would be needles. "You all right?" I whispered.

"Now. Yeah." At once, he was my teenager and my baby again.

I had never been able to let my babies cry it out. I'd never believed in it, resisting vehemently what the judgy mothers and famous all-knowing pediatricians suggested. When my boys were newborns and I knew less than nothing about what kind of parent I hoped to be, I had one certainty that guided me through the fright of being awakened by their cries and rushing to their teary calls of "Mama" — my babies did not have to cry.

I wasn't being a contrarian to the pediatric wisdom of sleep theory — there is no rebel spirit in me. I was driven by the visceral reaction I had. I couldn't bear the wrench across my middle, the actual cramping response to the sound of their unhappiness. I could literally feel their cries for attention or hunger or because the blankets came off. I had the ability to make it better, so I was going to do that. The attitude of this judgy tech was nothing new … All the you're-going-to-be-doing-his-laundry-when-he's-forty comments didn't touch me. Not comforting my kid sure as hell wasn't going to start when he was fifteen.

"It's gonna be okay, A-man. We can do this." I watched the moment happening to us. *This shouldn't be happening to us.* It was surreal. No one I knew was having a day like this. No one I knew had been through anything like this. It was a made-for-television movie scene, starring me. "I'm right here. Look at me over here. I'll be behind the glass," I said, as Aaron turned onto his back and someone laid the lead blankets across his torso. He wiped his face with his sleeve. "It's not safe for me out here. You get that, right?" The brown eyes stared. No nod, nothing. The same eyes that implored me as an infant begged me to make it stop now. It ripped my guts out. I backed away, and the machine started to move over him. I could hear small sniffles until the machine consumed him, whirring too loudly for me to make out any sounds. I would stand sentry until he no longer needed me.

I called Rick after dropping the boys at their schools. "Dr. Tobin wants to see me without Aaron. It can only be bad news. Otherwise she would have waited until the follow-up appointment when the results of *all* the tests are in."

"You don't know it's something bad and anyway you can't change the outcome by worrying about it now, so just wait and see what the doctor has to say." That was Rick. *Just don't worry.* His unemotional approach to problems put me in mind of *The Bob Newhart Show,* and the way Newhart's fictional Chicago psychologist would listen patiently to a client's anguished complaint and then bark, "Stop it!" The barking tone wasn't Rick, but the matter-of-fact belief that every person possessed a worry switch that could be turned on or off, or ideally, dismantled entirely — *that* was my engineer husband, but I was already in hyperdrive, my native terrain. For me, an information junky raised by a mother trained as a nurse, who brought medical cases and the words of dying patients to our dinner table, I knew only research could keep me calm until I saw the pediatrician the next day.

I remembered my hairdresser's words: "Aaron has acromegaly. You know, gigantism." This time, I couldn't just push them away. I couldn't close the laptop. Instead, that night I opened it and dove down the Google rabbit hole.

3

RESEARCHER

Research was a natural retreat for me; a non-fiction writer's safe place is annotating, cataloguing, and compiling. But I wasn't just gaining knowledge about gigantism, a disease I'd vaguely heard of — this was me possibly forecasting my son's future. Our lives. These were lines I would rather not untangle.

Gigantism? No way. I'm totally overreacting. Aren't I?

I clicked on the images this time, remembering how over-whelmed I'd been with the symptom lists and medical jargon the other time I'd searched. My mouth dropped. Beyond the Guinness Book of World Records illustrations and the photos of pus-filled tumours and teeth growing from extraneous body parts, there were clinical pictures, the ones staged to disguise identity but show the patient entirely. I couldn't stop staring. In fact I magnified to peer closely at the rows of faces. In many, black rectangles shaded the eyes of barely clothed children. There were adult men and women of various ages, a vaguely recognizable or famous face or two, dated black-and-white shots and before-and-after pairs. The after faces featured bent and misshapen noses, protruding jaws and cheekbones, the skin stretched tightly as if wrapped over too-small frames, like those pale-pink Silly Putty images that as kids we lifted from comic-book frames then stretched out of proportion for our amusement. There were pictures of massive hands splayed across people's chests, showing fleshy backs and sausage fingers. Was Dr. Tobin going to tell me this was happening to *my* boy? *If he has gigantism, what else is happening in his body at this very moment?*

I learned that gigantism is the disease resulting from a secreting pituitary tumour, which has its impact prior to puberty, and thus people diagnosed with it experience extreme height in their childhood or teens. Acromegaly is the outcome of the same tumour, diagnosed in adults, those of post-pubescent age. Gigantism sufferers are giants or gigantics. Those with acromegaly are acromegalics.

More mouse clicks and up popped a movie starring an actor with facial disfigurements caused by acromegaly. I read the description of his character: hideous face, insane, crazy about murder, on a rampage. It was called *The Brute Man* — Brute? My boy was no brute. On the IMDb site, I read the tagline for a film called *The Monster Maker*: "A mad scientist injects his enemies with an acromegaly virus, causing them to become hideously deformed." *Dear God, is this what Aaron might be facing, living in a world where he's viewed as a monster?* Still more searches found Richard Kiel, famous for his role as the killer Jaws in Bond movies; Ted Cassidy, the actor who played Lurch on the *Addams Family*; and other actors including Rondo Hatton, Fred Gwynne, Carel Struycken, and Eddie Carmel. All of them men who portrayed villains, or menaces, whose size or appearance was used to intimidate and even scare. And there were a couple of pro basketball players I couldn't name, with the exception of Yao Ming, who I knew about from my avid sports-fan sons — who had been treated for a brain tumour.

A brain tumour?
A brain tumour.
A brain tumour!

André Roussimoff, otherwise known as André the Giant of wrestling and film fame, featured on virtually every site, as did Tanya Angus, a young American woman in her twenties living with acromegaly. Her before-and-after photos were startling. At twenty-one, Tanya appeared of average size and height, athletically built, posing for a shot in a bathing suit. Just five years later, she was a foot taller and nearly three hundred pounds. She was about seven feet tall now, close to four hundred pounds, and she needed a walker for support. I peered into her eyes on the screen, looking around and through the bending bones and thickened features caused by uncontrolled levels of growth hormone. *Who's baby are you, sweetheart?* I kept reading about Tanya, even after there was nothing new. I heard her interviews. I smiled when she smiled. She was magnetic. I wondered if I could bear to watch the documentary about her, with its terrible, sensationalized title, *Help, I'm Becoming a Giant.* Then I saw her with her mother. Neither of them had any privacy anymore.

My mouse-clicking pace raced. I feverishly searched *gigantism* and *life expectancy* and came across an excerpt from a medical paper that said giants' bodies are always in proportion, a distinguishing feature. Then I read that rapid growth means that giants usually die at a young age.

This frightening search led me to the heart-rending clip from Billy Crystal's 1998 movie, *My Giant*, where he says, "You've never seen an old giant, have you?"

This isn't happening. I hurried through the kitchen to the place on the coffee-coloured wall where we marked the boys' heights. I saw Aaron's latest mark, far above those made each February on his birthday the years before. I held a ruler against the wall. He'd grown almost five inches per year for three years. Was that the kind of rapid growth the articles mentioned? It was faster than his brother, but there was a two-year age difference. *Growth spurts are a normal teenager thing, aren't they?* Was time being stolen from him now? Had we been losing precious time for years? Had I rationalized so much about Aaron's appearance, complaints, pains, and idiosyncrasies that I didn't know what was true anymore? Had I taken so long to get him to a doctor that his life was at risk?

This cannot be happening. There is no way this long shot is happening to my kid. I practised this self-talk in an effort to still my racing heart, but a tight band had constricted around my middle. The nausea of despair joined it soon after. That whisper emerged from the recesses where inner wails wait — the same mantra I'd heard earlier, pealing in a tone I couldn't recognize because it was more animal than mine: *Please, not my baby ... please, not my baby ...*

I shuffled down that same hall behind Dr. Tobin, past the height chart and the weigh scale and the adorable murals, my own dead man walking. She hefted the test results onto the desk as I took a chair across from her.

"It's gigantism, isn't it?" I said. It was time to say it out loud.

Dr. Tobin pursed her lips. "I'm afraid it is. Although the CT scan was incomplete on Friday, and we need an MRI to be absolutely certain, I wanted you to know it confirmed a large mass on Aaron's pituitary gland."

"A tumour."

"Yes, a tumour."

I have no idea how long I stayed in the office or what happened after that. If I made follow-up plans or promised to update her, wrote something down, and on what, I don't know. I remember none of it. All I could picture was a tumour, a sinister red bloody blob, and the euphemism *mass* did nothing to dilute the fixation.

Dr. Tobin escorted me to the office door and stayed with me through the hallway, past turning heads of waiting patients. She must have known I was on the verge of a meltdown and didn't want me getting hysterical in front of mommies about to walk their sick wee ones into the exam room. I remember looking back and seeing her wet blue eyes, and managing, "What do I do now?"

"Keep the appointment you have tomorrow with the endocrinologist. It's good timing," she said as I stepped on the elevator.

I bolted for my car and once inside I pulled myself into a quaking, wailing ball. A big *X* had been drawn over my boy's name. Someone else was getting the last-minute reprieve that should have been mine. My kid had a 3.6 centimetre tumour in the middle of his head. How did we go from sore knees to a brain tumour? The wall of images fanned across my mind, screen captures from my internet search the night before. The sullen faces, distorted bones, bent hands, and massive feet, movie monsters, incredibly tall men cast in sideshows. It was a terrible mosaic of my boy's future.

I called Rick. "Do we tell Aaron now? Do we tell him at all? Should we wait until we know more?"

We tossed the good-parenting options back and forth like a football on fire. "This one isn't in the Parenting Handbook," he tried to joke.

"He knew something was wrong. Even before we did." I reminded Rick of the night less than a month before when I'd picked Aaron up from my parents' house. He loved to hang out with my dad, whether working on some DIY project in the basement workshop or watching sports on television, chips or red licorice and a can of pop in hand. When I got there, my mother met me at the door.

"I gave Aaron some Tylenol," she announced, mild disapproval on her face. "I hope that was okay with you."

"Why?" I asked her.

"He had a headache. He says he has them *all* the time and that he's been telling you, but you don't do anything about it. I think you better look into this, Patti."

I brushed past both her and the accusation. I was used to those from my mother. Aaron was stretched out on a blue recliner in the living room, sharing a bowl of something crunchy with my father. "Another headache, A-man? Is that the first one today?" Aaron was flushed, a little worked up, something I could read from his expression but also in the tight grip he had on the arm of the chair. *Why is he upset?*

"First *today*." And then he added, more snarly than plaintive, "Mom, I *swear* there is *something* in my head."

Where did that come from?

"Okay, bud. Let's talk about it while we drive." I was not having this conversation in front of my parents for a whole bunch of reasons. My mother, who was extremely knowledgeable about severe medical conditions after years as a surgical nurse and then a palliative-care worker, had been an alarmist when I hadn't inflated each sniffle into pneumonia when Aaron was a little guy. I wasn't about to expose Aaron or myself to what I knew was the probable outcome. She'd make me feel like an incompetent parent for not investigating this suspicion fully. And I would do anything to avoid conflict with my parents. There'd been too much of it. We weren't the kind of family that talked about things, despite what my mother liked people to believe. And they weren't *those* kinds of parents or grandparents, who would step in and do absolutely anything to help if something was really wrong. Whatever was up with my boy that night, or any night, I knew we'd be dealing with it on our own.

He'd thought there was something in his head. And there was. There is. He was right. Why hadn't I done something then?

We'd talked about the headaches, but I'd tried to downplay their seriousness, normalize them for Aaron. He was really sensitive to health matters around that time, and I wondered if he was more likely to consider medical extremes because two of his school friends were seriously ill. Randy was in the hospital in the late stages of metastatic cancer. Kirk had been experiencing grand mal seizures, his epilepsy having taken a severe turn. Aaron had been the kid who called for help on the football field and stood by Kirk during a seizure not long before. This explained the urgency and maybe even his tone; he was rattled, and I wondered if my parents had fanned his paranoia a little.

"Could it be cancer?" Rick asked me.

"It's unlikely, from what I've read." Then there was silence. "How much should I tell him?" I was thinking out loud. "He has the right to know everything. He's almost sixteen. Can he handle this?"

"What are you gonna say?" Rick asked.

"Only that they've found it, I'm thinking. You know Aaron, he's anxious enough. I won't tell him anything unless we know for sure. I'm afraid he'll go from hearing the word *tumour* to thinking he's dying."

"Okay. You'll know how to handle it. I'll see you at home right after. I'll get out of here early. You'll find the words, you're good at that." And he was back to work. As ever, Rick was supportive of me to the extreme, even though my friends would often comment that he left the most harrowing tasks to me. It was how we did things. And yet there were all those boxes stacking up in the garage that I was giving a wide berth to, holding my breath that I could keep their truth from the boys a while longer, and I was on my way to meet a realtor.

4

MESSENGER

I decided not to tell Aaron the diagnosis, opting not to name this phantom menace, and with that I'd spare him its rarity and the implications for a little while. Surely that was a reasonable approach.

It wasn't like I could ask someone who'd been through this. I sought platitudes for comfort: I'd know the right moment. I knew my child best and would do what was right. I was his mother, after all. My heart would guide me.

Clichés are right as much as they're wrong. I was pretty certain there hadn't been a platitude invented for this one.

I headed for Aaron's school, thankful I'd have a chance to tell him about the tumour before we went to get Justin, whose dismissal was later in the day. There was a drop-off loop at each of the boy's schools. Usually, I read a magazine, knit a little, did a crossword, or used that time for list-making, my compulsion and passion. Now I sat frozen, eyes fixed on the blank page of the notebook in my lap.

The bell went and kids poured out the school doors. I stared into the rear-view mirror. There was no time for a dry run and the words weren't coming anyway. Maybe I could just get out of the car and run, keep running until they found me cowering under shrubs in someone's backyard. Not likely. I was the adult, the parent. The thing Aaron would need to get through this.

I had to swallow repeatedly to keep the nausea from rising into my throat. I clenched and unclenched my fists around the steering wheel. *Some support I'm going to be.* He needed to know — because I couldn't justify not telling him and because our relationship was founded on us always telling the unvarnished truth. Among the promises I made to my sons was not to sugarcoat things. Turned out crap homework? Let your job slide during a hockey game? Made one of those proverbial bad choices all teenage boys make? I always let them know. That road ran both ways; it was one of our deals, and Rick and I enforced reciprocity.

Could I carry this for him? Should I? I sat in my car rationalizing how this might be a mistake, how medical mistakes happen all the time, so why scare him? I tried to convince myself that maybe my motherly responsibility was really to *not* tell him. If I never said it, it wouldn't be happening, right?

Aaron's rust-coloured anorak appeared out of the glass doors behind my car. He would have looked like all the other boys, with their backward baseball caps — his royal blue and sporting the bold white horseshoe logo of the Indianapolis Colts — their baggy low-slung jeans, high-cut sneakers, heavy backpacks, and the ever-present hoodies, except he was about a foot taller. Aaron walked with a little limp, his knees still so sore even though he'd been excused from gym class for over a week. He was with a boy I didn't know and they were laughing together. He was so happy. I was about to take that from him.

He yanked open the back door and tossed his bag in, saying "Hey, Mom," and closed it again, hard. Flopping down into the front seat beside me, he yelled, "See ya," to the kids gathered on the sidewalk, awaiting their rides. He swung his long legs inside and fastened his seatbelt. *What should I do, drive away? Tell him here? What if I get us into a car accident?* I hadn't put the car in gear, which drew his attention. I was paralyzed, still flexing my fingers around the steering wheel, staring straight ahead.

"What?" he said.

And I just blurted it, knowing I'd be tossing a live grenade into the tenderest spot in the universe.

"I saw Dr. Tobin today. She got the CT scan results."

"Yeah? What is it?" Watery dark eyes and pale cheeks with reddened blotches turned toward me.

"It's a tumour."

Pulled the pin. Released the spoon. Ten. Nine. Eight …

Aaron exploded. His fists flew. He punched his legs. He pounded the dashboard and shook his head from side to side as if he was trying to loosen a swarm of bees. Then he stared hard at me, tears streaking his face, shouting, "Nooo! No, Mommy! No, Mommy!" Shock had reduced my teen to a toddler. I saw the hands on the clock rotating backward, taking away time, stealing his present. He hadn't called me *Mommy* in years. I felt like my brain was going to burst out of my head. I couldn't bear to look at him, but I couldn't look away. I had no right to be exempt from this. If he had to bear it, so did I. Wind rushed by my ears. White noise. There was only his pleading, his begging, "Why, why, why me?" I hadn't dared to move the car yet, my own vision blurred by tears. High-school kids sauntered by, looking into the car. Aaron was raking the skin on his face with his fingertips, head thrown back against the headrest. "I knew it. I just knew it. I knew something like this would happen to me. I knew it, Mom."

I didn't have any more words. He'd heard enough from me. I rested my right hand on his leg, offering it to him, and bowed my head. I didn't know how to bear that his world was crashing in around him while I sat there doing nothing, doing this *to* him. I was failing him.

Justin noticed the tense quiet in the car when Aaron and I picked him up at school right afterward. We exchanged looks in the rear-view mirror. Aaron didn't turn to acknowledge his brother when Justin got into the back seat; Justin knew better than to ask. Little brothers are masterful readers of body language. It's a survival skill. *Don't rankle your brother* was a script Justin read from well. I tried to offer the usual banter with my younger son but my best attempts at after-school small talk must have been lame. Telling Justin that his brother had a brain tumour was going to be nearly as difficult as telling Aaron had been, but that would have to wait.

What the hell are we supposed to do next? I felt like I was hovering over a gimballed map table, the horizon line where sea meets sky lit only by my kerosene lantern, my nervous fingers running across an ancient, tattered sea chart to rest on the dark patch that deterred sailors of old from the unthinkable — the ornate beasts of unsailed waters. *Thar Be Dragons.*

Back home, Aaron flew through the front door and stomped upstairs to his room. I trailed after him. Leaning against the door frame, I fumbled out, "I'm sorry." It was all I had. His back was to me where he lay curled in the fetal position, the way he slept because he was otherwise too long for his queen-sized bed. *What should I do now?* I couldn't perch casually on the edge of his Toronto Maple Leafs bedspread and pull him to me in a hug, as I would have years before. This was his space and he deserved his privacy. While I was ready for him to talk, cry, scream, or even punch, I knew I had to let him take the lead. Whatever I was going through, that was mine. I couldn't feel what he felt.

I busied myself in the laundry room next door to his bedroom, pulling the boys' brightly coloured T-shirts from the dryer and suspending them on hangers from the drying rack. We'd been so pleased to find school gym clothes in Aaron's sizes at the beginning of the year. The XXL burgundy-and-gold shirts and long, loose basketball-style shorts in an XL were such a comfort for him. He hated when clothes emphasized his shape or drew attention to his height. My tears were stymied by a smile that took over my face when I saw my dresses hanging beside Aaron's T-shirts: the same length and half as wide. I loved his size, loved him just as he was.

I went to the kitchen and started dinner, even though it felt like desertion. We had to eat. I was mindlessly pulling things from the fridge, chopping vegetables, careful not to lop off a finger in my state of upset. *Wouldn't that just be perfect?* But the thought of it helped me hold my emotions together.

Dissolving right there in the kitchen would have signalled to both boys that the figurative house was on fire. They had never seen me cry. Maybe a drizzle of happy tears or when I was really upset by my mother, but they'd never seen me break down, and I *really* wanted to break down. But nothing had changed yet for Justin. I did feel some relief at that. *He can go on still believing he's safe, can't he?* Maybe nothing had to change for him. *Do I have to tell him?* It seemed only fair that he be left outside the bubble where Aaron and I were now trapped, for as long as possible. *Why bring someone you love into hell with you?* I could offer one of my boys sanctuary a little while longer, surely. And I suspected Aaron might not want his brother to know. It had happened before when Rick or I inadvertently shared information too freely. Justin had been furious when I told Aaron he had detention for something. It wasn't about what he'd gotten in trouble for. Justin said, "It's that Aaron will bug the crap out of me, like he's never done anything wrong, because he's sooo freakin' perfect." Likewise, we'd had to be tight-lipped during the most recent hockey season when Aaron's team lost a particularly high-stakes game and he loudly and firmly told us we were *not* to tell his brother about the "disaster of a game."

But the tension this night was palpable. There was no music playing, no homework at the kitchen table, and no Aaron talking to me or nagging at Justin to go out to the backyard rink and shoot pucks until dinner. I wondered how long it would be before I'd have to tell Justin what was going on. *Who am I protecting — him or me?*

Justin came up from the basement when I called him for dinner. By then Aaron had come down to the kitchen and stretched out across two pressback chairs, still hiding his face behind his bent arm. We couldn't ignore the sniffling.

"What's wrong with *him*?" Justin said, pointing at his brother, who was just a few feet away.

No reaction from the chairs, so I said, "Aaron got some bad news today. Just give him some space."

"He already takes up enough space, doesn't he?"

"Not today, Jay. Please?"

We all looked at the phone when it rang the first time. When I saw my mother's number on the display, I was tempted not to answer. "Aaron, it's Nana. Can she know?" I asked him, glancing at Justin. Aaron didn't move or uncover his face, he just burst with, "No! I don't want anyone to know. I wish you didn't even have to tell Justin. Everybody will be all, 'How are you?'" — said with a nasally, pitying voice — "and I can't say I'm okay. I'm never gonna be okay again. They'll just feel sorry for me and I hate that." Justin stared at me wide-eyed.

I sighed and picked up the phone. "Hi, Mom."

"Are we going to see Aaron on his birthday?" she asked. His birthday was a few days away. "I know we're not important or anything. But our oldest grandson *is* turning sixteen and it would be *nice* if his parents could make sure his grandparents got to see him."

I knew that my mother would take the opportunity of Aaron's diagnosis to do the "I told you so," pouring salt into the deep gash that my guilt had slit across my gut already. I didn't need her to know yet. I needed time to bolster my courage to confront her. I knew that paradoxically, my mother would find a way to downplay the seriousness of the tumour — she'd tell me about someone she'd looked after who was *much* sicker or she'd blow it off, saying that the doctors were assholes and didn't know what they were talking about because she'd never heard of such a thing — because this wasn't cancer, her specialty. To her, nobody was really sick unless it was the big C. It wouldn't matter that it was her daughter facing the news, that her grandson was suffering. She considered herself an expert on shocking prognoses, and granted, she did have thirty years of experience. She could always produce the most extreme medical tale, with herself at its centre. This disease was outside everyone's scope. I got off the call as quickly as I could, deferring birthday planning to my sister, Kelly.

After the boys were in bed — Justin, sensing the seriousness of whatever was going on, didn't press for any more explanations — I violated Aaron's wishes and emailed Kelly and my brother, Jeff. We weren't in the habit of regular chats, and news blasts were rare. My sister, who was seven years old than me, and her husband, both high-school teachers, lived in a nearby town with their girls. We made sure we got together for all the family occasions, the kids' birthdays, Nana's and Poppa's birthdays, and Thanksgiving, Easter, and Christmas. The cousins were nearly as close as siblings. Jeff and my sister-in-law lived a long day's drive away in Maryland. They had a ten-year-old daughter, Hunter, whom we saw once a year. I remember telling Kelly and Jeff to "hug your kids" in that email. Kelly would be hosting Aaron's birthday party for my family. I asked her not to ask Aaron how he was doing when she saw him; we needed to wait for him to out the news.

Kelly and I always made the extra effort to be the back-up parent for each other's kids when they were young, doing pick-ups for each other and being the first choice for babysitting.

Having aunt status was important to each of us. Kelly had her children after I had Aaron and Justin, so she had years to dote on the boys. Their infant and toddler milestones were as memorable for her as they were for me, and she took the news about Aaron's health very hard.

"I'll do anything to help," she promised me, sniffling. "And I won't say anything to anybody if Aaron doesn't want me to."

Aaron's moods and his reactions had always been central to our family dynamic. We had a saying when the boys were young: *If Aaron isn't happy, nobody's happy.* His mood had always been a predictor of either peace or needing to walk on eggshells in the house. Big guy, big personality, Rick and I had always agreed. It seemed inevitable that I was going to set him off somehow. Telling the news or not telling the news. Staying nearby but not getting in his face about it. Busying myself with his brother, cooking, or the house. I was in eggshell territory — hell, I was walking on flames. I'd have to manage Aaron's reactions, harkening back to the days when I had two handsy little preschoolers grabbing things off grocery-store shelves. I didn't want to make this worse for him. I didn't even know what worse would look like.

I retreated to the internet, and that night in the dark I would find the press release that connected me to Dr. Graham — the kind, Los Angeles–based endocrinologist who, the day after our phone call, emailed me two names of experts who had trained at the California hospital with him and who practised near us, in Toronto now. If only having the names was the essential last step before having the comfort of expert care. I had to figure a way to get Aaron in to see the doctors on that list.

5

ADVOCATE

Aaron's leg bounced like a jackhammer against mine, and he yattered loudly about school, the NHL, how he wanted to get new shoes ("Mine just aren't pure white anymore"), what he would be eating at McDonald's after all this ("I'm ordering one of everything on the menu"), and why there was only news on the overhead television, implying (not very subtly) that adults are all morons to care about the day's headlines. He didn't want a response from me, and I didn't try to get a word in lest I got fire-tipped arrows from him in return. I needed him to co-operate with the appointments and tests, and this meant play small, tread lightly.

I sat in a darkened corner of a pediatric cardiologist's exam room while an all-business physician placed sticky electrodes on Aaron's bare chest. We'd waited only four days since Dr. Tobin's referral for the appointment that would typically have taken months to get. It was happening after regular office hours, and the cardiologist was running the portable ECG machine himself.

Aaron was tense, choosing to stare at the ceiling rather than look at the man who leaned across him to run leads back to the monitor. Watching the sinus rhythm reminded me of how many times I'd stood at my father's bedside wondering how his heart managed to keep on beating. Aaron blurted one-word responses to the doctor's questions for a few minutes but finally just said, "Ask *her*," nodding toward me. I hoped that his pediatric specialty would give the doctor a heightened tolerance for belligerence.

The ECG complete, Dr. Noonan removed the electrodes gently, then paused to rest his hand on Aaron's shoulder. Aaron looked up at him at last. Dr. Noonan bent toward him a little and said, "Even though you're big, that heart isn't going to let you down." And turning to gesture at me, he added, "and neither is that woman. Whatever you have ahead of you, *she* is what's going to get you through."

I welled up with tears. The doctor's comment had tossed a pail of grey paint on the elephant in the room and admonished Aaron as I couldn't have. Normally I would've taken exception to someone calling out my child, but it was deserved and done like a compassionate father who happened to be a doctor. I credited that moment, which Aaron and I never spoke of, with his adjusted behaviour at later visits with specialists.

A few days after the cardiology appointment, I returned the delicate Dr. Kirsch's warm smile when she shook my hand after greeting Aaron, and her petite frame kept me smiling for many minutes after. Another tiny-statured children's specialist examining my oversized boy. I wished I could share this with someone. She was fine featured with dark-brown eyes and tightly curled almost-black hair. Dr. Kirsch's specialty was the endocrine system — the hormonal implications of Aaron's tumour.

"The CT scan revealed a 3.6 centimetre pituitary adenoma," Dr. Kirsch read from the report, something we did not need to hear again. "I'm so sorry," she said. "We're going to need to do a lot more blood work to screen for hormone levels."

We spent well over an hour in a consultation room that barely held three chairs and an orange upholstered examination table with six grey metal drawers beneath. A roll of fresh white paper was suspended under the vinyl headrest, which was decorated with stickers shaped like teeny sparkly, rainbow-striped umbrellas. *Is it someone's job to put the stickers on there?* Dr. Kirsch wanted medical histories, Rick's, mine, and those of our immediate and extended families, everything back a generation or two. None of it seemed connected, but I answered the questions.

Aaron was antsy, but attentive. If I missed a detail, he reminded me. His memory was incredible, and he loved to show it off, even when that meant showing someone else up, typically me or Justin. He was slouched way down in his chair, teenager I-don't-care style, and I wanted to poke him to tell him to sit up straight but didn't have the heart to nag.

"Is he allergic to anything?" Dr. Kirsch asked.

"We wouldn't know," I said. "Aaron's never even taken cold medicine, let alone an antibiotic." He'd had surgery as an infant and the antibiotics had been dosed while he was under anesthesia then. Nothing since.

She looked up from her notes. "Are you serious?" I was.

More questions. Recurring ear or throat infections? Surgeries? Other hospitalizations? Was Aaron injury prone? I had no idea why she would need to know, and it was quite a test to come up with details long lost, like how Aaron chipped the tip of his elbow when he was three. But he was happy to tell the story of slipping down the wooden basement stairs at his grandma's house, adding, "I put on *quite* the dramatic show! They shoulda thanked me, really. It was Thanksgiving too." Dr. Kirsch giggled with him.

"Has he always been tall?" she asked me. I told her that he had always been in the 95th percentile or more. "Let's check his height today," she suggested, asking Aaron to follow her into the hall. Another child was standing poker straight, arms like rigid swords at his side while a nurse announced his "four foot two," and marked it on her folder. The little boy's mouth fell open when his wide eyes locked on Aaron walking toward the measuring stick on the wall, and he blurted, "Wow. How tall is *he?*"

The nurse in the pastel-pink scrubs ushered the boy away. "Looks like he's gonna find out just like you did." I heard the examining room door click behind them. It took an extra wooden ruler and the use of a step stool for Dr. Kirsch to determine that, at six foot five, Aaron was in the 99th percentile for sixteen-year-old boys.

Three twentysomething nurses, all sporting similar versions of loose-fitting pastel scrubs and Crocs, watched. (*Do they shop together?*) It was comical to see Aaron's doctor measuring him, hand on his shoulder for support as she leaned across him, resting his chart flat on his thick brown hair to ensure accuracy. It was a time before smartphones, or mine would have been clicking pictures madly.

I pulled a couple of school photos of Aaron and Justin from my purse, and Dr. Kirsch looked closely at them then stapled them neatly to her folder's inside cover.

"Are your high-cut running shoes comfortable for you, and what size do you wear?" she asked Aaron.

"They're the only thing I feel stable in and they're a fourteen. I turn my ankle a lot without them. I do better in skates than shoes." Dr. Kirsch was hitting on so many details. If I'd considered them together, the way she was doing, I might have raised an earlier alarm. And I was the one struggling to get him up for school when he was exhausted from a rotten night's sleep, seeing how he'd sweat on his pillowcase, giving him Tylenol more and more frequently for his headaches, and buying the expensive leather high-top shoes that were so difficult to find once his size went beyond a thirteen. *Why hadn't I been alarmed when Aaron outgrew his shoes so quickly or when the height markings on the kitchen wall jumped up by multiple inches instead of fractions of an inch like Justin's?* I wondered if Dr. Kirsch could see the tears stinging my eyes or sense the mother's guilt building up inside me as I listened to my boy describe how he'd felt sick to his stomach a lot lately. He told Dr. Kirsch about severe cramps in the morning, the pain he felt walking any distance, and being so hungry all the time but dreading that he'd feel nauseated after eating. *How had I not noticed how crappy my son was feeling?*

Dr. Kirsch shifted in her rolling chair to face Aaron and me.

"Are you an anxious person, Aaron?"

Aaron shrugged. "I guess I am. I sweat all the time, even when it's cold out. I'm always hot. I take an extra shirt with me everywhere, for when I sweat through. Mom keeps one in her car. I get really nervous, like coming here in the car today. Ask my mom, I never shut up, cause I'm so nervous." He'd proven his own point.

Dr. Kirsch examined him. "Don't move your eyes or your head, keep looking at my nose." She extended her arm at shoulder height, formed a fist, and pointed her index finger. She slowly moved her arm to bring her finger toward Aaron and asked him to say *now* when he was able to see it. She repeated the action from the right and left, above and below, for each eye. I'd never seen this done before and never been through it myself. I'd learn later that this innocuous little test, which seemed both casual and completely subjective, helped her conclude that Aaron was beginning to have peripheral vision loss.

"Stand up again, then bend from the waist." She ran her small hands up either side of his spine. "His back is perfect," she said, turning to me. *Oh, good, he doesn't have scoliosis. Too bad about that pesky brain tumour.* She took Aaron's blood pressure and temperature. Her eventual report noted that Aaron had hypertension and peripheral vision "field cuts," but she didn't say that to us.

"Let's do a bone age while you're here," Dr. Kirsch suggested.

He barely protested having X-rays taken of his hands, unlike just days before when he'd refused to leave the car to have his knees X-rayed. Returning to her office, she asked Aaron to lift down a heavy black volume from a wall shelf. Aaron and I were fascinated by this massive cloth-bound book containing hundreds of X-rays of hands, with tiny handwritten measurements overlaid on the dark spaces between the finger, thumb, and wrist bones. It was so analogue. The process was simple: Compare Aaron's X-ray measurements of the dark spaces between the epiphyses, the hardening (ossifying) ends of the bone — to one of the reference images. Aaron's bone age was fourteen years and four months, nearly two years less than his actual age.

"His growth plates aren't closing," Dr. Kirsch said. *Whatever the hell that means.* She punched a couple of keys on a calculator, then looked up at me. "Aaron could keep growing until he's seven feet four inches, plus some usual puberty growth," she said, as if telling me they wouldn't be providing lunch on this flight.

"Well, that can't happen," fell out of my mouth. I didn't even take a breath. It wasn't a desperate mother's wish for a miracle. It was a manifesto, a battle cry. *What will his health be like at that height if there are so many problems now?* This made no sense to me. Aaron was growing taller but his body wasn't maturing? I had so many questions but I couldn't ask them in front of Aaron. I knew I'd need to research how that worked but I was wrapped up in the horror that my son could be seven and a half feet tall, another foot taller than he stood now. Height had just become the most prominent feature in my kid's life.

Marking the boys' heights on the wall at our house was something we loved doing; height was neither a concern nor noteworthy. We measured everyone, adding marks for the dog, Grandpa, and even the boys' buddies. Rick and I were marked on there too, leading to the kids' teasing that over time our marks were going to get lower on the wall as we shrank "like all old people do." We used a butcher's knife to do it, which made the kids squirm, and might have been why Rick and I liked doing it so much. Resting the knife's flat blade on their heads would press their hair down enough to get some accuracy as we pushed the knife point into the drywall. Sometimes we tapped the knife handle with a hammer, just for effect. I'd looked at the sum of inches the night of my internet search, but I hadn't had a reason to consider the timing of the growth. Even how much Aaron had shot up in the last three years wasn't necessarily worrying; I'd known boys Aaron played hockey with who had sprouted rapidly between novice and peewee divisions. Above-average height was in the family too. Rick, my dad, and my brother, Jeff, were all six feet tall, and Rick would have been taller, but he'd had steroid medication in his childhood to treat a nephrotic condition, which constrained his growth. When Aaron was a year old, Dr. Tobin had projected that he would be six foot six and about 210 pounds. She later calculated that Justin would be six foot three and about 180 pounds in adulthood. All that fuelled my multi-layered rationalizations. I'd thought he was on track. But I didn't consider that boys typically don't stop growing at sixteen. Aaron could have three or four years of growth still ahead of him.

Dr. Kirsch listed off the other tests we should have done. "And a twenty-four-hour urine collection and a glucose tolerance test ..." I dreaded the one that required Aaron to fast in advance. The kid could barely go an hour without food. We would see Dr. Kirsch again a week later to go over results. The priority was to start the referral process to get Aaron seen by a neurosurgeon at the Hospital for Sick Children in Toronto, the country's top pediatric hospital. The tumour had to be removed. "That could take months," she said. "But I'm guessing when SickKids sees his diagnosis and my report, they'll schedule him faster than that."

This wasn't the first mention of surgery, and I'd read some about that as well. It was logical that if a tumour was causing him to grow, removing it could stop the growth. There was likely a lot more to it, but that was how I wrapped my tired, worried brain around it that day. I was taking it all in, leaving no space for fear. I didn't know how Aaron was feeling about hearing all of this. I glanced down at the sheet of paper Dr. Kirsch had been taking notes on during our session and it was an unorganized smattering of teeny illegible words. It reminded me of how we tossed metal shavings on paper in high school physics class when we were learning about magnetism. "I'll write the referral today," she told me. *Would anyone be able to read the thing?* "Is there anything else we need to talk about today, Aaron?"

Aaron piped up. "Can ya make my guts not feel sick all the time?"

"I sure can," she said, and she began scribbling away on her prescription pad, sheet after sheet. "I'll give you instructions for how to add these slowly," she said, passing me the stack. "I think it's a good idea to get started right away, even before we see another set of blood work. It's quite likely he'll always need medication after this." There were four prescriptions. My son who had never taken even an antibiotic now needed instructions for his daily medication regimen.

6

WEIGHTLIFTER

In less than a month, I'd taken Aaron in to talk about sore knees and somehow we'd seen three pediatric specialists and done many tests. It was record time in my experience (or anyone else's I knew) in our publicly-funded provincial health-care system. I was grateful and more than that, amazed, when I heard a voicemail later that day from the neurosurgery department at the country's top pediatric hospital offering us an appointment in a week's time. Alarm bells were sounding in my head, revving my adrenalin, turning me into a high-speed automaton. Calendars, lists, copies of referral letters, and confirmation letters were piling up on my bedside table.

Denial had left the building.

Some disquieting conflict within me had taken its place. I believed that if I gave in to my instinct to immerse myself, embracing this worst-case scenario as our reality too quickly, I'd release forever the long-shot hope that Aaron could somehow be spared. If I accepted that the flying monkeys were circling, was I failing my son? Wasn't ceaseless, boundless, even absurd faith what I owed him as a mother? I wasn't sure how to be what he needed now; I just knew sitting still with blinders on wasn't going to cut it.

I shared some information very sparingly with my two closest girlfriends, Val and Dana. Talking about what we were facing and trying to keep them updated (given the supersonic speed of information coming at me) was often more upsetting than helpful. And talking about it meant that I'd hear how dire the medical situation was too, as it was coming out of my own mouth. I was telling Rick everything, but it was always cut into bite-sized pieces so that the kids wouldn't hear. I emailed him links as I learned more about the disease, but I never knew if he followed through and read the information. We didn't have that kind of relationship anymore.

Avoiding talking about it became my way of keeping a foot in the waters of disavowal. I had to live this, and making lists, recording numbers, and taking notes were the preoccupations that made it possible. When I met my friends' sympathetic gazes across the table in Starbucks, or heard their *Holy shit! How can that be?* that gave way to *How the hell are you keeping it together?* — I'd wonder too. I didn't know how I was doing. I was doing Dory: I just kept swimming. I'd lost my ability to be in the moment, hell-bent instead on growing armour around myself so that every time someone asked during a hug, "How are you?" I wouldn't collapse into tears and wail about the injustice that this was happening to *my* child. I felt so exposed. I hated feeling out of control of my emotions and by default, my dignity.

Jan, one of the trainers at the service-dog charity, randomly hugged me one day and over my shoulder whispered, "How ya holdin' up, mom?" The cracking voice that erupted from my throat was only vaguely recognizable as my own. Against any will I could muster, I blurted, "I'm not," and when she pulled back to look into my face, I was already in the middle of an ugly cry. I'd never had a personal conversation with Jan before. It had been all dog commands with her. How the hell was I going to keep it together with the hockey coach, schoolteachers, and other well-intentioned people, who by now had heard that one of the Hall kids was sick? I cautiously shared what little information I had with a few others, with predictable results: murmurs of placating statements from fellow puppy raisers at Reef's service-dog classes, and reassurances from anyone else who had caught wind of what we were going through, like the boys' teammates, although all they knew was he was tall and there was a tumour. "He'll be okay." "He's so healthy." "I'm sure it won't turn out to be serious." "The tests will rule everything out." "I heard of something like this before and it was nothing in the end." That was what I wanted to hear, but those people hadn't seen the test results, the specialists' faces, or the speed at which doctors were making ASAP and STAT referrals and requests for my kid. Other people, Rick included, hadn't done the internet searches, didn't know that Aaron had ten or more symptoms of gigantism, didn't know about the shortened life expectancy or the pain from being too large for your own skeleton and organs. I was keeping it to myself unless someone asked. That way, I didn't have to hear it. I was split down the middle, not wanting to be irrationally hopeful nor give up believing it might all be an elaborate coincidence. But indecision wasn't going to find Aaron a brain surgeon. And all those people weren't going to walk beside me while I did.

When Aaron was diagnosed, Val followed the process closely, even though I was pulling away. Then she called me one day when I was downtown at the hospital with Aaron, and with her classic no-bullshit stance, laid it on me: "You can shove everyone else to the side and suffer alone, but when you bleed, I bleed, and I'm going all the way with you on this. Don't you fucking dare treat me like everyone else." My blinders were on, and even her tough love couldn't get me to raise my gaze.

Happier down in the medical weeds than looking at my son's strained face, I kept researching and delved into information on cause. There was virtually nothing.

"Is this genetic?" I'd asked Dr. Kirsch.

"There is some new research saying it's possible," she told me and offered to have Aaron's genetic material collected and banked for him at the Hospital for Sick Children. That way, if testing his DNA became necessary to cross-reference against genetic research results later, this blood could be a diagnostic marker. Aaron signed the forms himself, saying, "If this will help someone else someday, I want to do it." Then he asked, "Will there be another needle though?"

As a family, we talked as little as possible about medical stuff in front of the boys. That meant that Justin couldn't glean much, a few words at the table or whatever he overheard on my cellphone calls, but he remained part of what was happening to his brother through annoying behaviour, poking the bear. I hadn't considered the possible repercussions of the steady flow of information. Tensions are high when teenagers go head to head anyway, but now new issues bubbled beneath the surface in our home. There was more haggling over who got more of something; brotherly teasing sometimes turned into cutting words that tore too deeply.

A freak warm spell was turning the ice rink in the back-yard into a small lake. I'd seen the boys through the large kitchen windows, lobbing clumps of slushy snow into the inches of water accumulating within the rink's boarded frame. Kids and puddles, an unfailing pairing. It was only a matter of time before a snow fight broke out. I was so glad to see them hanging out.

Then: "You suck, Aaron." (The boys entered the mudroom.)

"Screw you, Justin. I *can't* run. It hurts." (Closet door slam.)

"You're just running inside because I'm faster and you know

it," Justin yelled back. They spilled into the kitchen, shoving at each other, Aaron's wet socks flopping loosely over his toes, Justin's boots tracking slush onto the floor.

"Hey, hey, guys. Knock it off! And boots, Justin," I said. He stepped back onto the tile in the mudroom, yanked his boots off, and tossed them across the room in the general vicinity of the drying rack.

"Charming," I said.

Aaron was sitting in one of two armchairs at the window, wrapping a hand-knit throw around his shoulders. Justin stormed over and threw himself in the other armchair. He was intent on pursuing this.

"If Mom wasn't here, I'd put you in your place, you runt," Aaron threatened before Justin could start again.

"Yeah? Well, you might be bigger, but at least I can run."

"I *can* run —" Aaron started to say, then leaned back in the chair and pulled the blanket over his head. It wasn't true; Aaron couldn't run. Not anymore. Not without extreme pain.

I saw the difference in their heights, well over a foot, and just over two years apart in age.

"You're right, Jay, he really can't run like he used to," I said.

"I know. He's *so* slow," Justin said. *Give me strength.*

"That's not what I mean," I said. "I mean he can't run because of the disease. Aaron has really sore knees. He hurts all the time. Imagine if it hurt to run. You wouldn't do it either, even for your pain-in-the-neck little brother." He listened, maybe even saw some sense in it. (It was a high-risk proposition speaking teenage boy to their faces.) "Running is just not something his body can handle anymore."

Justin fell quiet. And Justin was *never* quiet. Classic second born, he was all action, very little forethought, but predictably pensive after the fact. He'd been spending a lot of time in his room instead of hanging out in the tall chairs at the kitchen breakfast bar, demanding snacks and asking his usual torrent of questions. We were coming undone, each in our own way.

I hadn't sat on the edge of the boys' beds at bedtime in years. It had been ages since the three of us, and sometimes the four of us, stretched out on one of our beds while I read *Harry Potter* aloud (doing all the voices) or spun stories for them, like the ones about Sgt. Redwing Blackbird, which I'd promised to turn into a kids' book series.

Justin had taken off upstairs after the harsh words with his brother, tossed his wet clothes in a smelly heap, and crawled under the covers.

"What, Mom?" he said when he saw me perched at the foot of his bed.

"Let's talk about what's going on with your brother."

"I don't care, Mom, he's ... he's so ..."

"Yeah, I know he is." We both laughed.

I'd thought it was business as usual for Justin. Unfortunately, I was doling out information to him in the same piecemeal fashion I was receiving it, keeping the medical stuff on the down low, without noticing the effect it had on him. Sometimes, I'd tell him about a doctor's appointment or offer up a morsel about one of Aaron's symptoms, like his sweating or the reason for his headaches, or warn him about the possibility of surgery. Justin listened with genuine interest, but his emotional reactions were flat, as if I was telling him a story about some stranger's illness. Why hadn't I noticed that he just didn't seem to be putting all the pieces together?

"He's really sick," I told him now.

Justin smirked. "I'll say he's sick!" *No shit, Sherlock.*

"No, seriously. Aaron's disease is really scary. Even I don't know enough about it yet. We still need to find a doctor who's worked with a kid like Aaron."

The smirk disappeared. "Will he be okay?"

"He's going to get even taller, like I told you," I said.

And now a hopeful glance. "That's okay, though, right? Being tall is cool."

"Sure, except that a person can be *too* tall. So tall that they have problems like they can't walk very well or their legs and backs get bent, and it's really hard on their hearts to pump blood to that big body."

"Aaron walks okay." A touch of defiance.

"For now, Jay. For now."

"Will he be able to run after they operate on him?"

"I don't know. We don't even know of a surgeon that's done one of these operations yet. I'm still trying to learn about it all."

"You *have* to find one, Mom. You have to find someone to help Aaron." Now Justin's eyes were as worried as my own.

Until just a few years before, I'd still strolled through my boys' rooms at night before I laid my own head down. As a nervous new mom to a preemie, I'd done this from the first day of Aaron's life, compulsively checking on him, making sure he was breathing. The boys didn't know I still did it; I'm not even sure Rick knew. They might have been a tad old for it, in someone else's eyes, but at least I wasn't crawling on my hands and knees up to the side of their beds listening to their breathing like in the kid's storybook *Love You Forever*. Actually, I had done exactly that, but I'd graduated to tiptoeing in to pull blankets over them and finally to a simple glance from the door.

That night, stricken and suspended in the flotsam of my overwhelm, I went to Justin's and Aaron's doors and looked in. I wished it was a decade earlier and I could crawl in beside them without them waking in alarm. I wished I could wrap us in a single family-sized life preserver so the inbound rogue wave would have to take us all if it sought one of us.

I wondered if Aaron was processing all of this like I was. Was that ever-present sense of invincibility that teens seem to possess protecting him from letting this all sink in?

I dreaded being alone in the car with him. What was I going to say if he wanted to talk about it? After each appointment we went to McDonald's or Subway, and as we ordered, I felt the weight of the latest information descend on me. *Why the hell doesn't Rick have to handle this?* He might even tell Aaron the wrong thing, still figuring it out himself. And there *was* no one else. If anyone was going to screw up, it must be me because I'd never forgive someone for having a negative impact on my boy's health.

Taking on Aaron's health crisis meant I had less time for my own care. I wasn't on the phone to my girlfriends, and I wasn't seeking out comfort. My refuge was writing — the one place I'd ever felt safe, unjudged. I ran screaming to my journal some days, hoping the words that had been forming into sentences in my mind would lay themselves down onto the page. More than that, I needed to see I wasn't crazy.

An acquaintance suggested, not unkindly, that looking after myself needed to be paramount. *Don't say it. Don't say it.* On cue she trotted out the cliché: "You're no good to Aaron if you don't look after yourself, inside and out." *Yeah, right. Like I'm going to take a spa day.* If I felt like hiding, never seeing anyone, never telling the story or crying in front of people or hearing my self-pitying voice again, Aaron must have felt the same way.

1

WRECKING BALL

We only talk about timing when it's bad. And this was bad. It couldn't have been worse. I was carrying the weight of a massive secret, one about to spill all over my boys' lives.

The lawyers had been hired and paid. The paperwork, lists, and cheques had changed hands. The steady accumulation of boxes in the garage marked what I'd be taking out of our home, our life, this marriage.

In near screenplay timing, after close to a year of tense but largely amicable and confidential negotiating over email, Rick and I had agreed that once I found a house of my own, we would announce our separation to Aaron and Justin. I'd signed the papers for a new place. In a cruel twist, I'd signed them the day I met with Dr. Tobin and learned about the tumour. We could not have foreseen that the timing of our separation would coincide with this other worst thing to ever happen to our family, Aaron's diagnosis. I feel strongly now that we would have done things differently if the legal separation, custody arrangements, and financials hadn't been signed and notarized when we learned what our boy would be facing. But hindsight is a kick in the ass.

I'd bought the house.

We'd separated our bank accounts.

It was done.

Nothing about negotiating the end of a marriage could be called simple, nor should it be. No one ever got married with the intention that it would end or that they would go willingly into the dissolution. We surely didn't. But Rick and I did the best we could, negotiating what we both felt was fair. More than anything material or emotional, we dreaded the conversation with the boys. *That* conversation — the delusion-destroying moment we outed the facade to our beloveds. I'm sure we both felt shame taking an invaluable scaffold out from under our boys. We both understood that once the children knew, there was no going back, no peering over our shoulders with doubt, because their hearts would be in the mix. We'd always put the boys above everything, and unfortunately, above the marriage that had made them. That was what we did wrong.

The plan was to put it to the boys as shared custody, but in practical terms, they would spend more time with me because I was the designated homework-help parent and Rick travelled so much for work. The boys and I would be leaving the big country house we all loved so much and moving into the town where Aaron went to high school. Without Dad.

I was physically and emotionally overwhelmed, but I confined the signs of it to my room. The beginning of a dangerous habit for me. I'd started going to bed early, waking only when the alarm blared the next day. My stomach churned with anxiety when I was awake, and my mind spun with worries, lists, and numbers I couldn't organize as I attempted to figure out how to orchestrate life without Rick. Now there was Aaron's medical stuff too.

I was going to have to manage everything on my own: mortgage, bills, car payments, house repairs, and all that owning a home entailed. A single parent. I didn't know if the kids would turn on me, refuse to leave, or worse. I remember my friend Jill telling me her little daughter took off running out of the house, down the road, and into the woods when she and her ex-husband made their announcement. They'd had to call the police to help in the search.

Rick and I had exchanged numerous emails on how we wanted the conversation with the dudes to go: simple; no blame on either of us; make it clear this had nothing to do with them. I wanted them to know their dad and I would remain the friends we'd always been and that we intended to parent them side by side just like we always had, but from two homes now. I knew Rick would step in when I faltered, but I also knew, as with all things of an emotional nature, I was going to have to lead this talk.

I looked at Rick; his eyes were full of tears as he sat on the edge of an antique pressback chair, legs outstretched, ankles crossed, clenched hands wedged between his thighs. An oil painting of an English harbour — a wedding present — above his head. I raised my eyebrows to ask if I should start.

"Boys, come downstairs," Rick called up to their rooms. We watched as Aaron and Justin settled themselves into chairs opposite us at the table.

"What?" Aaron asked, seeing our strained expressions.

I took a deep breath. "Dad and I need to talk to you guys."

"Nooo!" Aaron bellowed, the sound one makes crowning the hill of the roller coaster. "What now?"

Another deep breath. "You know how Dad and I don't really do anything together anymore?"

"Oh, no," Aaron blurted. He knew what was coming. Justin did not.

"Well, we think it's time we tried living in separate houses."

We all looked at each other. The boys waited, eyes wide, mouths open. My tears dribbled.

Aaron spoke first. "Who will we live with?"

"Me," I said. "Well, both of us. You'll go back and forth or something." Silence again. I filled it with, "We'll work it out. I bought a big house for us in town."

"Will there be high-speed internet?" Justin asked and we all laughed. The slow dial-up connection in the country house had always been a source of consternation to my tech-savvy younger son.

"Pretty traumatized by the news, huh, buddy?" Rick said, keeping us laughing.

"The speed is so bad here," Justin said flatly.

"Well, I guess so," I said.

"When do we move?" Aaron asked.

"April," I told him. Just weeks away. And that was that. The boys headed for the kitchen and rifled through the snack bin while Rick and I sat waiting for the worst to come, certain they'd be back with questions, outrage, grief. We had talked about how to handle the blowback. I read everything I could online. We'd put off telling them because of what was about to hit us. My heart raced. Rick's knee bounced.

But the boys never came back to the room. Rick and I sat in the dining room together, staring at the hardwood floor through our tears. After I heard them go up the stairs, my eyes cast around the room into the spaces I knew so well because I wiped them, decorated them, shifted our lives within the contours of these bones. This was our dream house, filled with the cherry-wood floors Rick had laid himself and antiques we'd collected throughout our eighteen years of marriage. The Big Blue House — everyone in the area called it that — got its name because it looked like a replica of the denim-blue house with the huge round window in its second storey rendered iconic by the kids' television show *The Bear in the Big Blue House*. That window was my porthole; the house, my vessel. I insisted on using female pronouns for the house, which stood sentry on the knoll, permitting no one access to the ten acres of forest behind *my* home. In my master's thesis, I'd explored how nature is essential to forming place attachment. A sense of place and my life at Big Blue embodied that. The forest surrounding my beautiful country home was the setting for my meditation in motion, my *waldeinsamkeit* — the feeling of being alone in the woods. It names a sensation we all recognize, one I'd had in the five acres around my childhood home, an awareness as real to me as the consciousness of my own skin, the taste of my breath. Rick had maintained trails for me on the property, which I walked daily with the dogs and often the kids. Leaving the forest was a metaphor for tearing away from Rick and loosening the deeply woven intention my heart had to be with him forever. I knew the trees on sight, the rocks that stuck up under the moss in certain places on the path, the soft peat where the dogs took the corners too fast, and the places where the thorny branches grew and caught the flesh on my shins in the spring. Robbed of the familiarity, of the forest, and of his comfort, I was coming unmoored. And I couldn't process the emotional upheaval because Aaron needed me now. I would never get over the loss of that place, of him. My soul would grieve it forever.

It still does.

If we had told the boys earlier, would it have changed anything? What if we'd told them before that CT scan? Would we still be together? And, what if the diagnosis had come before we were sure it was over?

I brought the gavel down on myself. I could never let myself ask that question again. And I haven't. I replaced the questions with a permanent ownership of what happpened; the shame of being the one who chose to end it is my dark cloak.

As terrified as I was of being without Rick, I wasn't paralyzed — quite the opposite. Whatever I may have been, I couldn't be any longer. In a flash I was no longer a wife, because the mother calling was bigger than everything. I'd asked for the divorce. That was on me. I couldn't lean into Rick now. Aaron had to face forward into the murk, so I had to face this. I wanted to run into Rick's arms, beg to start again, press myself against him, but it simply wasn't fair. None of this was fair. I rowed on. Without a partner, when I needed one most, I forced myself to live with this choice, like so many others.

Did anything matter — even our marriage — when we had a sick child and were only just coming to understand the extent of his illness? We couldn't deal with all of it at once, and Aaron needed us to be on top of everything. There was nothing that didn't pale in comparison.

We would have to feel our sorrow and loss later.

I knew firsts without Rick would be the worst for me. He'd been my shield with my family, diverting pain-causing attention and bearing witness to the insults of hellish family dinners. I decided to have Aaron's sixteenth birthday celebration with my side of the family and not invite Rick. I couldn't separate from the man and still rely so heavily on him. I loved him. I would always love him, but I had to quit Rick, cold turkey. More than anything, I was scared of being in the world without this person I trusted so completely. In retrospect, it may have been my encounter with a monster worse than being alone — Aaron's diagnosis — that made me stop leaning on my husband. Or it was shame, plain and simple.

I tasted that bitter pill when I had to tell my dad, nearly the only person in my life who'd ever shown a genuine interest in me. I'd walk to his small printshop after school when I was a young girl, usually finding him behind a noisy printing press or bindery equipment. He always had his hands full of something heavy or inky. No matter what was being printed, cut, scored, punched, or folded, he would hit the Stop button when I pulled on his pant leg or came into his view behind a machine. He made me feel like what I had to say mattered, something in short supply in my young life. He was always excited to see me, calling me "Toot" or "Spike" or some of the other nicknames he used for me my entire life.

In the lobby after a hockey playoff game one evening, Dad and I waited together while Justin got changed. Over hot dogs and coffee (I suspected the food was more than half the reason he never missed a game!), I told him the latest news.

"It's looking like surgery is likely. It's the only treatment that might actually cure Aaron, but I don't know if he's a candidate yet. It's still too soon to know if they can remove his tumour. It's really big."

"Do they know whether the tumour is cancerous though? Can they figure that out?"

"It's almost never cancer," I told him. "The disease is caused by a tumour that secretes growth hormone." I hoped that made some sense. "Dad, we finally told the boys that we're separating."

"Christ! You're having a helluva week, aren't ya?" he said, squeezing my arm. Dad sighed. "Your mother and I have always liked Rick, you know that; he's like a son to us. But we don't have to live with him ... or with you for that matter!" He grinned, hoping to lighten the mood, then sighed again. "I just wish it was different for the boys."

"Me too."

We'd been hiding our separation from the world for long enough. We'd attended all the boys' sports banquets and team parties, games, and events until then, and although each of us might have begged out of the occasional tense family gathering, now that the boys knew, we (make that, I) would have to face the explaining. "Where's Rick?" would become the standard greeting I got whenever I arrived everywhere. It was my walk of shame.

As Aaron's birthday approached, we kept our promise, in this and in all negotiations, to talk about it and not make assumptions. We knew that if one thing went awry, if one of us harboured unmanageable hurt or felt taken advantage of on a single point, financial or otherwise, our amicable pact would implode, and us with it.

"Are you sure you don't want me at the party? If you want me to, I will. You know that," Rick said.

I really do. I really do. "Thanks, but I guess I've gotta handle it sooner or later," I heard myself say. *Please come, please come. Puh-lease say you aren't ready to not be included in my family dinners. I can't do this.*

"Why isn't Dad coming?" Justin asked, when I told the boys about the party arrangement.

"Because it's time I faced the music." This was likely the day Justin started discreetly watching how I was doing from his increasingly silent perch.

A week later, Aaron sat on the beige brick fireplace hearth, his long legs sticking straight out into the middle of the room. Kelly and her husband, Ray, my nieces, Laura and Michelle, and Nana and Poppa had been stepping over those legs all day. Justin and the cousins lounged nearby on the floor like a litter of wriggling puppies. The moment arrived.

"Aaron wants to tell everyone something," I announced.

Kelly turned the volume down on the television and everyone turned to look at him. "The doctors figured out what's causing my headaches," he said, hands clasped in a prayer position, wedged between his bouncing thighs. Silence. "I have a tumour." I bit down on my lip and covered my face with my open hand as tears dripped into my lap. Not a word from anyone for seconds. I couldn't take my eyes off of him.

Kelly jumped in. "I'm sure the doctors will know what to do."

"I'm sure everything will be fine," Nana soothed. "I knew someone who had a brain tumour and after surgery he was right as rain."

I looked over at Poppa, clad in his characteristic plaid flannel shirt, his own long legs crossed, thickly socked feet in sheepskin slippers. His rocking chair had stilled. His eyes leaked tears and his chin quivered as he reached into his pants pocket and pulled out a pristine folded white handkerchief. Aaron was my father's special friend, the first grandchild. He'd had two and a half years to be grandfather to one little boy, and Aaron's birth had made him the happiest he'd ever been in his life — he told me that the day he arrived home from an airshow in Oshkosh, Wisconsin, with the only souvenir he'd bothered to buy: a little flight jacket for his grandson, A-man. Rick and I had hurried to have a child after our marriage because of my father's life-threatening heart disease. Aaron's birth was widely understood to be a gift, a piece of legacy insurance for Poppa.

Dad wept silently. No one said anything else. No one comforted anyone. I wasn't surprised. We were more the kind of family that hurls verbal barbs than pleasantries, "barracudas with nail polish," as one of my high-school friends once called us. Like a collection of little green army "mans" (the boys' childhood terminology), we held our positions, frozen until it was time for the next scene.

Finally, someone lit the big *1* and *6* candles on the cake. Someone else cut it, passed the plates, and I don't think we ever sang "Happy Birthday." I let myself wonder what Aaron's next birthday would look like, and if we'd all be together again. My nieces were teary when I told them about the separation. Justin played right along, like all was normal, but every time I glanced his way, I caught him looking at me. Everyone managed to eat cake and joke with my boys about how many pieces they had. The business of Hall family dinners resumed.

"You were amazing," I told Aaron on the drive home, hoping I'd neither insult nor enrage him. I might have been angry that no open support came that night for Aaron, but I had horrors to face and I'd never expected any member of my family to be by my side as I did it anyway, not even my father. I didn't have time to recruit my bannermen.

The next month was a clash of Aaron's intense medical needs and the closing period of the real-estate transaction. Taking care of the endless tests and appointments while packing a house, moving my children away from their father, and handling legal and financial matters was daunting. It was my money now, not ours, and I felt intense guilt that masked my grief. The boys still needed to get to and from school, hockey games, and practices. There were the animals and Reef's training. Rick and I diligently protected what normalcy we could and maintained the boys' calendar meticulously. I did not write. I read only medical material, added more boxes to the growing stack in the garage, and fell dead asleep at night on emotional autopilot, trying to suppress the relentless reminders that I was divorcing my husband, leaving myself without a partner, a best friend, a trusted confidante. Sleep was my only escape, but it came only after shivering and panic attacks that began plaguing me then.

"It's like I'm running a movie camera, up above on the crane, not walking the halls of hospitals," I told Lori, one of the warm-hearted trainers for Reef's service-dog charity. I raised my arms above my body and wiggled my fingers to convey the out-of-body experience.

"Maybe that's how you're coping," she said. "Trauma works that way, right? Like a small person after an accident can lift a car off someone being crushed by it."

I didn't feel traumatized. I felt lethargic and tired, sure, but not like an accident victim. I blankly watched my disembodied feet moving along hospital corridors, sometimes ancient and cracked terrazzo and other times ornate glossy pseudo-marble. I recorded the details, not feeling anything about them. I saw me glancing up for an information icon or ahead for a blue-smocked volunteer to ask for directions to the wing of the building that we needed. Aaron plodded along behind me, trusting me to get us where we had to go, uncomplaining. I manoeuvred monolithic buildings that felt either too austere or too commercial to be facilities for caregiving, and I made mental notes of how to get to certain clinics and labs because I knew that we would be coming here again. Perhaps more than once.

"You won't know how hard this has been until it's over," Lori said.

"The divorce or Aaron's health crisis?"

"Each of them. Both."

I watched Aaron and myself, trying to see us from a stranger's view. We were separate but obviously familiar; our relationship would be unclear from our body language. He didn't want affection or warmth from me on hospital days, just for me to respond to his requests and questions. I was guide, voice, and enforcer. He managed by maintaining whatever detachment he could from me. I accepted it. Cool as I was (and I was *freaking* cool), he was still a dude having to hang out with his forty-something mother.

I could relate. I avoided connection. The stress was like a lead blanket. I could be in tears at the smallest expression of caring, so I kept a layer of Plexiglas around myself. I was walking, talking, taking down names and numbers, office locations and hormone levels, all as if I were managing a project instead of a life-or-death personal mission. At what cost? I didn't care.

This wasn't numbness exactly; the sensation was more mechanical. One becomes accustomed, accepting what is because there doesn't seem to be any way to change things. The deluge of negative — as Aaron put it, "No one ever tells me I'm going to be all right" — inspired consistent defensiveness in me. I was ready for crisis at all times. I assumed that the worst was likely to come again and again. Blind optimism was not my landscape anymore. My feet left no impression on the floors, but each of the corridors and testing rooms left a mark on me.

As I watched the two of us from above, I wondered what we'd look like in two years, five years, or more. *Will we get "or more"?* Would Aaron remain youthful and strong or would the effects of the bone-bending, spine-straining, and soft-tissue massing take their toll? *When will there be canes and wheelchairs?* I had no way to know. I just kept putting one foot in front of the other.

My friend Dana and I had had a regular daily check-in for years. As two self-employed women, we'd often worked side by side in a coffee shop — before my travels for hospital visits. The texts determined where we would hole up with a couple of lattes to fill in the latest inspirational entrepreneur workbook or read up on the time-management system used by today's most successful self-employeds. They were also a mortality and sanity check. We did this for each other; we filled gaps left by our partners.

Dana and I met when our younger sons played lacrosse on the same team. After the obligatory ten-second handshake at the first game, our husbands had run out of things to say to one another, and Dana and I had filled the awkward silence gabbing about smelly sports equipment and living in a house full of men — perhaps as a means to avoid admitting out loud that each of us feared the violent nature of lacrosse and our boys playing it. Now our connection was not so much about our boys as our lives as single women.

The kids' schedules are INSANE today and I'm so stressed out, Dana texted. And she really was. But I couldn't relate anymore. My reply was something previously unimaginable, like Taking my kid to the brain surgeon. I didn't care that it might sound self-pitying, because it was pitiable. But there was no right way for Dana to respond.

My life had become ludicrous. I couldn't relate to my friends' everyday problems anymore. Other moms were worrying about curfews, making good choices, getting those dirty socks off the floor. Who had time for that shit when I had to figure out how to navigate my son through medication, surgery, and radiation. The surgery could be done through his nose, over his lip, or as a craniotomy, which meant splitting his head open like a pumpkin to scrape out the offending growth. The tumour had his pituitary gland surrounded and it might continue to secrete growth hormone unabated no matter what we flung at it (his levels were at thirty-seven times the average). The Master Gland might or might not do some of its jobs; Aaron's systems could be drowned in hormones, like testosterone, or robbed of others, like thyroxine. Each person's manifestation of symptoms was as unique as their hormonal composition. The variation of hormone levels was to blame for the physical extremes I'd seen online. I knew just enough to scare myself out of denial but not enough to know that I'd need to live in the landscape of the unimaginable once I learned what this disease could do to him.

This justified me pulling inward, becoming more private, leaning on others less. If anyone had tried to tug information from me, my shattered state of mind would have been obvious, like light cracking through a boarded-up window. But everyone asked about Aaron, and almost no one asked how I was doing anymore. Maybe everyone besides Dana and Val knew better than to ask me.

Rick and I just kept doing what we did so well: We parented our kids as a team. I passed on website links to him as I found them, and we spoke out of earshot of the kids about how much

Aaron really needed to know. We agreed that we would never tell Aaron what I knew about shortened life expectancy unless he deliberately asked exactly that question. Whether Aaron was researching on his own, I couldn't know. He said nothing on the subject and asked very little. I told him only what his doctors confirmed or what I found from experts with definitive opinions, careful to be brief and to the point. I hoped that he could face it in bite-sized pieces, but my dilemma was how to give my son information without rendering him too scared to live in his own body. Rick and I hoped that there would be an organic process of curiosity that would guide this. When Aaron really wanted to know more about data, symptoms, and heaven forbid, the prognosis, I would answer.

"I just want to feel better, Mom," he said to me after an appointment. "All these doctors and tests and days, and nobody can make me feel better. All they do is treat some invisible thing that I can't even tell is there, and still I feel crappy all the time." The attention was about his body, but not how unwell he felt, his "guts hurting" as he called it. I was so pleased that he had no idea of the scope of the problem and yet so very sad that he was dealing with nagging symptoms.

"Sometimes, I just wanna go, *Helllooo* ... I'm the one you're supposed to be helping," he said, "and looking at scans of my head is not making me feel better. Mom, why don't they stop talking to each other and ask me how I *feel?*"

He was right, of course. The long game was so horrible, and outgrowing his body would have such a deleterious effect on his life that medical attention was focused there. Meanwhile his headaches, joint pain, aching muscles, sleeplessness, sweats, and nausea persisted, and no doctor (not even those with a specialty that took up two lines of type on the door sign) was able to make him feel better.

8

BODYGUARD

The night before our appointment at the neurosurgery clinic, I helped Aaron with his homework, an assignment asking students to contemplate different careers and their future lives. We cut out photos from magazines of houses, suited men with briefcases, and marketing slogans for posh brands like Ferrari — "Only those who dare, truly live" — and arranged them on the panels of the white bristol board. The heaps of images represented my son's plans for his long, brilliant life, dreams that included a high-paying job, the big house on the water, a wife and kids, dogs and boats and cars and cottages. No canes, wheelchairs, or hospital gurneys in sight. Would imagining his future this way raise any dire thoughts in Aaron's mind? I braced for a flurry of questions to come, but Aaron doggedly scissored and glued away.

Then he looked up from the tear sheets. "I *am* wondering something," he said. "And don't start telling me about all that medical stuff, because I *don't* wanna know. Just tell me: How many other kids in the world have this?"

I hated not having an answer to the one thing that he was curious about. "I'd be guessing, A-man. I don't know. There aren't any lists or registries for people who have it. It's a fair question, but I don't know." I danced some more. "Most people don't get diagnosed when they're kids. Like you."

"So, basically, you're telling me I'm an anomaly?" he said, sounding accusing and angry. *Anomaly?* Where did he even hear that word? Even to my wordsmith mind it sounded like he meant *freak*, and its synonyms were no better: *odd, peculiar, incongruous, abnormal.* These weren't adjectives you ever wanted applied to your child; it was way worse hearing him use them on himself.

"We'll have to go straight to the surgeon after we drop your brother at school early tomorrow," I reminded him.

"Yeah, I know," he said. "I don't wanna go."

"I don't wanna go either, but how else will we find someone who can tell us about the tumour and what it might be doing to you?"

Aaron turned to me, a cold stare fixed on his face. "But I don't want to learn that everything I feel, my knees hurting, how tired I am, and how slow I'm moving, are all this disease."

"Why not?" I'd tried once to explain that other people with the disease felt the same symptoms, hoping he'd feel more ... was *normal* the right word?

"Because it'll get my hopes up, that someday I won't feel all this crap, and that day is never gonna come." He banged the scissors down. "I just want to feel better. But now I know I won't." He pushed his chair back and stalked out of the kitchen.

The irony was sickening. Aaron couldn't face dreaming because a rare disease had stolen his certainty in any kind of future. He finished that poster board the following day; months later, when he brought it home, I tucked it away, determined to protect his hopefulness until he was ready to dream again.

I found Aaron in the living room, where he shot me an angry look. "What am I going to SickKids for? Isn't there some doctor at our hospital I could see?"

"No, there isn't," I said. "This, uh, thing they think you have is really rare. There's no one at our hospital who's dealt with it before."

Truth was, there was only a handful of doctors in the entire world who'd treated a teenage patient with gigantism. I recalled turning back to Dr. Kirsch as we left her office: "Is it fair to say that in your career you'll never see more than one child with this disease?"

"Yes," she'd told me, "and of the hundreds of endocrinologists I know, none of them will ever see a case in their careers at all."

Now that I knew how crappy he was feeling, I wished we could have a real conversation about it, but that wasn't Aaron's choice. He used to be such a chatterbox who loved to gab about sports, clothes, and video games. Even on mundane topics he'd toss in a few grunts while passing through the kitchen, yell updates on school from the shower, or offer a news flash of something on television while digging for clean laundry on the closet floor. But Aaron wasn't talking much anymore.

"What are they gonna do to me at SickKids, anyway?" He was enunciating the consonants, another sign of anger.

"I don't know, A-man." I didn't want to lose a chance to keep him informed, but I didn't want to terrify him either. If I said too much or was wrong about what he'd experience, he wouldn't trust me later on.

"You mean, we're going down there and *you* don't even know what they're going to do to me?" he shouted, practically spitting.

How the hell am I supposed to know? I've never had a kid with a brain tumour before! Aaron was intentionally trying to push my buttons. Neither of us knew who to be. I couldn't manage to be angry at how he was speaking to me, and I accepted that he held me responsible. I was glad that Rick had agreed to join us for the consultation, hoping that I wouldn't feel so solo in this medical mess anymore.

I had high expectations going into our appointment at SickKids. Why wouldn't I? I'd heard the stories and met people who'd come away from their kid's treatment there with a glowing story of deep gratitude, in awe of the sensitive way the hospital treated their child and ameliorated their concerns. Aaron's friend was being treated for his seizure disorder there, and his mother told me how a dedicated team of global experts often consulted on his case via Skype.

"The hospital is giving my kid a future," she told me. I hadn't been swimming in the murky medical water for long, but I was incredibly hopeful that the fitful darting from place to place and topic to topic would quickly end at SickKids. I wasn't hoping for a miracle, counting on a mistake, nor was I on bended knee begging the universe to say it isn't so. Not anymore. I just wanted a doctor that looked neither horrified nor stupefied. Someone who perhaps rubbed their chin pensively with a bemused expression of welcome intellectual challenge. The good doctor would consider words carefully before blurting them and then offer, "Well, I've seen worse." I would even welcome, "There are still a lot of options for Aaron."

SickKids is a hospital where babies have tests using the tiniest of needles and miniaturized machines. It also boasts spaces dedicated to play in every waiting area. Rick, Aaron, and I walked its busy hallways, which were decidedly more animated than those in other hospitals we'd visited thanks to the masses of children walking or rolling the halls and clumped in waiting areas. I wouldn't have been surprised to see staff in clown suits. The place was tailored to keeping kids smiling.

The three of us walked through a bright, multi-storey central atrium where a newly constructed glass addition, crafted in hunter-green metal piping, met the former outside wall of an older brick building. It was an architectural achievement, merging a modern public face with an institutional classic. There were few hard surfaces or sharp edges in the common areas. Corners were curved, benches cushioned, and the green metal tube infrastructure arched in an almost tree-like skeleton within the greenhouse of suspended walkways that traversed the complex.

"Mom, look!" Aaron tipped his head toward adorable tots in their colourful hospital gowns, some with butterfly or tiger face paint and wearing brightly coloured hospital masks, all with strings of beads around their necks (a hospital program to mark procedures bravely completed), and tried not to stare at tubes coming from their noses or arms. He'd spent all of his elementary-school years in a Montessori classroom where mentoring younger students is part of the culture. Aaron adored little kids. These ones were clearly experiencing so much discomfort. I wondered how this seemed to him.

As we found our way to Neurosurgery, I glanced into every space, trying to imagine where counselling and comforting was happening. Would I ever get used to seeing other people's kids in pain? Would I become one of them, know some of these families, befriend some of these exhausted-looking moms? It was easy to see families and doctors in boardrooms because any nonclinical space was surrounded by glass looking out onto the sunlit atrium. My eyes met those of other parents. Once they had been new here too. My son was now a patient in this place where people got the worst news and begged for results to not be true — I was one of those parents in the eyes of other people now. *This is one club I wish I hadn't been invited to.*

I felt the heat rise in my face when I studied the doors along the Neurosurgery hallway. There were whole storage rooms for DNA and records. Aaron would be a vial, a file, a case, a statistic now.

Somewhere in SickKids I hoped there was also recovery beginning for suffering families. I needed to believe that somewhere, patients who had once been very ill were just kids again. If we had to be part of this, I needed Aaron to be one of those kids. If any place could cure him, I was certain it would be this place.

The staff members milling behind the massive circular nurses' station didn't even look at Aaron twice when I signed us in at Neurosurgery. *Wonderful. A great start. A kid who is taller than every adult in this building is no big deal here.* While we waited to be seen in a large examining room, a regular stream of people slowly passed by, occasionally stopping at the door to peer inside. I assumed they were checking whether the doctor had gotten to us yet.

After twenty minutes, a very slim, soft-spoken surgeon in a white coat buttoned all the way down the front stepped inside the exam room, accompanied by another doctor. Neither introduced himself. We were accustomed to appointments that began with one attending who was then joined by many fellows, interns, and students. The surgeon, Dr. Lindgren — I gleaned by reading his name tag — seated himself on a very short wooden chair, which meant he had to look up at Aaron, who sat with Rick on a low padded bench facing him, their knees uncomfortably pulled up toward their chests on the toddler furniture. The second doctor and I stood a few feet back, leaning on the wall adjacent to the washroom. The room was designed to comfort children, obviously, but children didn't come in my son's size. Everything seemed Alice-down-the-rabbit-hole out of proportion.

Dr. Lindgren fired the usual series of questions at Rick and me; I answered. This continued for at least ten minutes as a group of three young doctors slipped into the room. Again, there were no introductions, no attempt to level the playing field, no "Do you like sports, Aaron?" Just a bunch of doctors gawking. That made five white coats; seven of us looking into the face of a nervous boy. *Who's looking after the rest of the children on the Neurosurgery unit?*

The surgeon asked one of the doctors, "What are some of the symptoms that we should ask about here?" A young woman with square dark-rimmed glasses, her hands worrying at coins or keys in the pockets of her coat, listed them off: vision loss, facial changes, lower voice, enlarged fingers, sweating, and joint pain. Two more doctors entered the room whispering among themselves. More questions from the surgeon. At least twenty minutes more of show and tell.

Dr. Lindgren finally turned to me. "We'd like to examine Aaron."

Rick looked up to where I stood, seething. This roomful of children's medical experts in the finest pediatric hospital in the country had not yet addressed my son. More white coats crowded at the door, craning their necks to look around and over the others, trying to check out the anomaly. Someone out in the corridor or at the reception desk had clearly been spreading the word.

My voice quaked a little as I spoke up. "One of you can," I said, "and one of us comes."

"Of course," Dr. Lindgren answered and he nodded at his Number Two, who moved over to an examination table, shuffling the others aside to do so. At least he pulled a curtain around the table to create some privacy. Keeping the other white coats on the outside, Dr. Morgan finally introduced himself. He studied Aaron's hands on both sides, turning them back and forth like slabs of meat in a butcher shop. He produced calipers from his lab-coat pocket. They looked like a barbecue lighter with a clear plastic loop on the end, which closed around Aaron's baby finger and read the measurement in millimetres out loud. Aaron stepped on a scale, then stood against a chart on the wall, which produced the usual giggles because it stopped at six feet; someone pulled a little ruler out of their pocket and passed it, disembodied, behind the curtain.

"Note the tongue," Dr. Morgan said to his colleagues. *What about his tongue?* Aaron just sat still and stared into my face. I was breathing heavily, the warm blush rising to my face as I got more and more offended. But what could I do? Now Dr. Morgan looked at me and said, "We would like to examine Aaron under his clothes, to take some measurements."

What? The tumour is in his head. This is neurosurgery, right? No fucking way. I glared and said nothing, willing to hear his explanation. I wanted to deck the son of a bitch and get the hell out of there with my baby tucked under my arm. They wanted to measure his genitals. There was no way I was allowing it. Reacting to my silence, the young doctor added, "We need to assess his hormonal age, as we know that he has pan-hypopituitarism, including low testosterone."

"You already have that," I said.

He pressed his case. "An accurate assessment of the stage of puberty your son is at needs to be determined."

"This is neurosurgery. And *that* has been done." I'd found my voice, one with overtones of Mother Grizzly and the confidence of weeks of internet self-education fuelled by pure adrenalin. The white coats wouldn't be talking about my son's privates or measurements in the coffee room later. "He had a full examination two weeks ago with Dr. Kirsch, the pediatric endocrinologist who referred him here. You have that report. If you don't, I brought a copy."

Without waiting for a reaction, I motioned for Aaron to come with me. "We can be done now, A-man."

With the examination notes in front of him, Dr. Lindgren, the only doctor sitting, began his pronouncements from the little chair he'd never left. Brain surgeons must be medical royalty. Aaron sat down with Rick, who gripped him in a sideways hug. I wished I could busy my child with one of the bead-counting toys or the board books that sat abandoned on the red table beside him. I wished he didn't have to be here for this part.

"We have never seen a pituitary macroadenoma that secretes growth hormone at this level or that has grown to such a size, an estimated 3.6 centimetres," Dr. Lindgren said. *They really like to repeat the measurement.* "It is quite large and has extended into the sinus. Although we have never done this surgery on a tumour like this or of this size … we could try to operate. We have done similar procedures. We may be able to improve the prognosis."

Try? *Did he just offer to try brain surgery on my son?* This was the fantastic and near-miraculous option that the largest children's hospital in the world had to offer? They wanted to wing it, give it a go? *The hell they will.*

The fire roared up from my belly. I didn't know if I was screaming inside my head or if the shriek was coming out of me, and I didn't care. I'd come expecting a solution and what I got was a room jammed with curious onlookers at an Edwardian carnival.

"You could *try?*" I managed. Dr. Lindgren looked at me placidly, as if this was nothing new. *Is he kidding? Is this the best I can get for Aaron?*

It wasn't just the sense of defeat in that moment pressing down on me; my gut was churning because Dr. Lindgren had mentioned "improving the prognosis." Aaron was sure to ask me about that later, and I didn't feel equipped to even find the words to tell him that most giants don't live past the age of twenty-five. *Which is only nine years away.* Today was not the day for him to hear how little time he might have. I was hit with a trepidation I'd never felt before. I had a sensation like I'd been lifted off my feet and the space around me was moving too fast for me to stand still. Anxiety was building, diluting the voices to white noise. Every face in the room was pointed at me and I was ready to run like a spooked horse. Not without my rider.

Smiling now, the doctor said, "We might not have a bed large enough for him, so something would have to be done to accommodate him. We could borrow a bed from another hospital." *Are you kidding me, dude?*

I dug deep and in an instant flipped some switch in myself that took me from raging, anxiety-addled mother to deliberate, strategic advocate. The silence was getting heavy.

"Seriously?" I said, half-laughing.

"No. We really don't have a bed for a six-foot patient." More whispering.

"Six foot five," I corrected. "And I understand that. I mean about the surgery. . . . You would like to *try* your *first one* on Aaron?"

Dr. Lindgren nodded.

I looked at Rick. He was stone-faced. This was on me.

"We can't agree to that," I said. Rick and I hadn't discussed this. I could feel the shaking of nervousness starting in me. My voice was going to give me away by quavering. I was speaking for both of us, and there was a good chance Rick might contradict me right there or after, when we were alone. I was risking my own embarrassment, but my son would not be a surgical guinea pig.

I didn't know if we were any further ahead when we left SickKids. We took Aaron to Starbucks for a ginormous hot chocolate. He jammed a chocolate chip cookie the size of his head into his mouth in a couple of bites while I jotted down some notes.

"What do we do now?" Rick asked, peering into Aaron's face. "Whatever you want, pal."

My cellphone rang. It was a woman named Sarah from the SickKids Neurosurgery Department. "Are you Aaron's mother?"

"I am." I was baffled.

"I've been asked to see if Aaron could take an MRI appointment for later today."

"At SickKids?" Aaron wasn't even going to be a patient there. There was some communication mix-up, I figured. But I wasn't going to lose the opportunity to get the test done. Aaron's definitive diagnosis at that point was hinging on an incomplete CT scan done at a regional hospital. I played along. "At what time?"

"Well, as soon as you can get here, they could take him, actually." Nothing happened that fast. Had Aaron's need for an MRI turned into an emergency? "Dr. Lindgren thought you might still be in the area. I'll need to go over a screening form with you in order to confirm the appointment, if that's okay?"

She began the questions as the three of us walked back to the car. Queen Street was noisy, and I was dodging people, plugging my other ear with my index finger to block the sound of city traffic.

"Has he had a stroke, head trauma?"

"No." *Not yet, anyway.*

"Does he have any piercings, any metal staples or sutures from an injury or previous surgery?"

"No," I said, laughing a little.

"I know, I'm sorry, but I have to go through this list for the Imaging Department. How about a prosthesis or artificial limbs?"

"Also, no," I said. "The only thing Aaron has is a brain tumour and a mouth full of braces." The phone line was quiet a second longer than I expected.

"Oh, that's a problem," she said. "Metal braces?"

I stopped walking. *Of course they're metal braces. What the hell does she think they're made of?*

"Yeah, the regular kind, train tracks with the brackets and wire, cemented on," I replied.

"He can't even go into the MRI room with metal in his mouth."

My stomach clenched. Aaron had to get an MRI fast if we were going to get a surgeon to operate soon. "I'll have to see if we can get them off, I guess." I was thinking out loud. There was no time to ask Rick, and he would leave this to me anyway.

"Okay, Mrs. Hall. I'll let this appointment go. I have another one for him."

I jotted down a date and time, snapped my phone off, and made a beeline for Rick's truck, where I dialed the orthodontist's office. "I'm so sorry, but could you please interrupt the orthodontist? It's an emergency." I hardly recognized myself; I would never have done this before.

"I was hoping you could see Aaron later today. We have a problem," I said when he came on the line.

"Of course, I'll squeeze him in somewhere. Does he need to see me or a technician?"

"Well, you tell me," I said. "We need to take his braces off. We're at SickKids hospital and Aaron needs an MRI."

"Is everything all right? Is it a hockey injury?" The orthodontist was a hockey dad of teenagers himself, so it was a good guess. *He won't have heard this one before.* "No, he has a brain tumour. We just found out —"

"When can you be here?"

It took ten minutes to pop off braces that the kid had suffered with for two years. Aaron was thrilled, grinning at me from the dental chair.

"Well, I can't say I hate the tumour today, can I?" he said, almost skipping when we left the orthodontist's office. I fed him hamburgers and ice cream on the way home.

The second Justin got in the car after school that day Aaron announced loudly, "Look, Jay, I got my bullshit braces off today!"

"Spare me the language, please," I shot back from the driver's seat.

"Sorry, Mom, but today I don't care."

Alien forces were amassing, descending on me in unguarded moments: when the boys and I were just hanging out in front of the television, or grabbing food from their favourite sandwich shop, or indulging in our expensive habit for Lego City sets. I'd

take a break to pull together a snack, and yanking open the cut-
lery drawer for a cheese knife, I'd see a row of pill bottles, enemy
soldiers, each bearing notes for dosage in my fuchsia highlighter
lettering. Medical appointments speckled our family calendar;
our lives were being invaded and I couldn't stop it from happening. Did Aaron feel it too?

Rick supported me doing a wildly expensive splurge for
Aaron's birthday. It might have been guilt, since we'd just told
them about the separation, but it felt more like abject indulgence.
Neither of us was brave enough to say what we both thought:
What if the kid doesn't have another birthday?

One night out with the boys to an NHL game included four
great seats, Aaron wearing a custom-made XXLT Alex Ovechkin
Russian national team jersey, and feeding the kids any food they
wanted, including twenty-dollar sushi plates à la carte (for VIP
seats only). I don't remember where we sourced tickets, but I
know they cost us a thousand dollars. Instead of watching the
game that night, I never took my eyes off my son. He was oblivious to my attention, thankfully. The four of us split into sets of
two and swapped partners at the end of the periods so each kid
could take advantage of the best seats we'd ever had. *Will we ever
be able to do this with our boys again?*

Most people going through divorce don't want to be around
one another, even if they stick to the we'll-do-it-for-the-kids
line. Would Rick and I always get along well enough to do things
like this? We promised to try. And we had to be different from
other divorced couples — for medical stuff. For Aaron.

I remember nothing except the look on the boys' faces
every time we said "Sure!" to their high-cost (and unhealthy)
ideas including dinner at Gretzky's, a trip to the giant candy
store nearby, and pre-game appetizers and drinks in the exclu-
sive members-only lounge where three players on the injured
list autographed the back of the white Maple Leafs jersey I wore

while my boys giggled madly. It was guilt, it was therapy, it was a celebration that the four of us were, if not fully intact, at least not visibly responding to a distress call today. That night, we hung off the sides of the life raft together, Rick and I exchanging smiles and raised eyebrows as the boys gave us play-by-play highlights on the drive back to the Big Blue House. Rick had moved to the guest room in the basement months before, and we were no longer a couple in any sense, but for now, we would all still be under one roof. And we could do things mundane and elaborate as a foursome for just a while longer.

9

VIGILANTE

By April, our lives consisted of hospital days and non-hospital days. On hospital days Aaron plodded along at his own long-strided pace, staying just a foot or two in front of me, close enough that I almost tripped on his heels when our feet got out of sync. He navigated obstacles at ceiling height that the rest of us didn't notice, like the lit-up EXIT sign and those pointing to washrooms, elevators, and clinics. The ones fixed in place and not swinging from eyelets were particularly dangerous for Aaron. He'd push a door open by spreading his fingertips out and pressing at its very top corner, while his thigh hit the push bar that was at my waistline. The long bent arm of the hydraulic box might have taken out his eye if he wasn't paying attention. His hat could be knocked off by it, but he had this — his world — all figured out.

In the early hospital days he walked behind me through the innumerable institutional hallways, but once he knew the way, he liked to go ahead so that he could yank open the doors, push all the buttons, and grasp all handles for me. It was something he'd done as a little boy too. Some proof that our lessons in manners had paid off, maybe. Or he was just the kid who has to be in charge. More likely that. When I walked in front I could see where we were going; otherwise my only view was the big red wall of Aaron's back. Even at five foot six inches, I was easily shrouded behind my giant son. But back there, as he careened through crowds, I didn't have to see people stare at him. And they did stare. They didn't just glance up and then retrain their eyes on the floor. They looked at the baby-faced, nearly seven-foot-tall guy and ran their eyes up and down him, maybe to confirm they weren't imagining or that he wasn't in costume, on stilts, or being carried on someone's back. Maybe they thought some circus entertainers had come to cheer up the residents. Up and down again, back to me where I had come into view, up at him, repeat. I guess when someone's head is only a couple of inches from the ceiling, it draws attention. Everyone's attention. They couldn't help but look. But it hurt me. I didn't know what it was doing to him.

I had always been terrified of conflict, but now I was provoked into making eye contact with the staring people. I hoped my glare would draw their ogling back to me. Away from Aaron. In enclosed spaces like elevators and waiting rooms, folks softened a little. They stared but tried smiling in our direction, as if cognizant of their rudeness and preparing to meet Aaron's gaze if he looked up from his phone, computer, or book. Sometimes if I judged their intentions to be genuinely kind, I'd quell the tension by blurting out something friendly. But they weren't always kind. There were the whisperers and — these were the worst — gawkers who elbowed the person beside them and nodded toward Aaron so their friend wouldn't miss the show. There were also the pointers and the people who tried to take a selfie, sidling up near Aaron, aiming their phones up to their own face and then tipping them just enough to capture him in the frame. In elevators, the food court, and on the subway they were the worst of all. People weren't cruel 99 percent of the time, but they offered a horrifying study in human behaviour, and regular, blatant reminders of our societal obsession with difference.

I added a one-inch turquoise binder with a magnetic clasp to the stack of notebooks that I took with me everywhere. It held essential test results, referral letters, and a cheat sheet of locations and phone numbers of doctor's offices and labs. I really could have used a smartphone back then. I started keeping a Word document with dates, measurements, weights, and hormone levels, not only because I couldn't remember — my brain was rapidly turning to mush — but because I'd already learned that passing it to the person creating a new chart or doing a pre-consult for the next specialist could achieve Priority One: minimizing Aaron's frustration. I didn't want us bickering about accuracy in front of someone. I didn't want us to be that pain-in-the-ass family that grouses in the office while the doctor is trying to get to the important facts. I knew that my diligence on this front worked because the follow-up letters sent from one specialist to another described Aaron as a "polite young man" and a "well-mannered teenager." They were more likely to make recommendations quickly and go out of their way for that kind of child (and his congenial, well-informed mother) and I needed that tactical edge.

And we were becoming good entertainment too. We were developing a bit of a schtick, with the comedic timing of a pair who'd done stand up together for a long time.

"How tall is he?" a stranger or new doctor, nurse, or lab technician would ask me (almost never addressing him).

"Six six or so," I'd say. (Audible gasp.) That was his height in the early medical days but the second digit changed to seven, eight, nine, ten, and finally eleven in time.

"Will he get any bigger?"

"Yup, he's still growing."

Then to Aaron, they might say, "Do ya play basketball?"

"Only if you're a Raptors recruiter." He had a vast repertoire of responses. My personal favourite was "No, I'm a jockey." That always left them with their mouths hanging open, and the delay while they figured out the size humour gave us time to make our escape.

We knew how to tailor our material to the audience — whether they were little kids, groups of teens, kindly older people, or name-tagged hospital personnel — and to the particular look on the face of the gawking person. We could meet the rude, demeaning ones right where they stood. These ones would often look at Aaron and then more than a foot down at me and ask, "How'd he get so tall?"

I'd be the straight man. "He's a giant. Like, André the Giant."

"How'd that happen?" the person might then ask, as if inspired by some movie plot about alien babies or gigantic man-eating plant pods.

"I was breastfed," Aaron would lob in. Poker-faced, we'd both step off the elevator, then giggle our heads off as we sauntered down another hospital corridor.

Keeping us fun together was easy. It always had been. And so little was left unchanged that we clung to the goofiness and humour that was the bedrock of our connection, me and my boys.

Meanwhile, I ran battlefield-scale manoeuvres in my mind while I went about my daily life. I had to be doing something related to Aaron's medical situation all the time. A backward glance now shows me that my intentional exertions weren't always what moved things along; sometimes it was chance. I would research random medical references I saw dropped in online stories, and then the universe (another comedienne) would plop the solution in my lap. I was too deeply imbedded to recognize that coincidences were opening up treatment options more quickly than anything else. Meanwhile, these evidences of providence confirmed the six degrees of separation rule. You know the theory, that if you could map out your network, you'd find you were a handful of steps removed from knowing someone like Queen Elizabeth. Actually, it has a more logarithmic basis, and it's about how humans are all connected by our social relationships. It wasn't a theory to me anymore.

One of the first twists of fate showed itself back at SickKids, after Dr. Lindgren admitted that his team didn't have a surgeon who had performed a transsphenoidal procedure — the removal of tumour fragments using instruments and a camera inserted through the nostrils. So I asked if there was even a surgeon in the entire city that had seen one of these.

"Yes, there is, at St. Michael's Hospital. Cusimano does these."

I gasped. "Cusimano." *It couldn't be the same one.* "Michael Cusimano?"

"You know of him?" Dr. Lindgren asked, surprised I presume, that I was tapped into brain surgeon 4-1-1.

"I actually do," I said, feeling the amazement at the same time I was saying it. "He's my father's doctor," I said. "Or he was. He cared for my father through a head injury years ago."

Michael Cusimano had been the on-call neurosurgeon after Dad was T-boned in a car accident years before and barely survived injuries to his head and one leg. I'd never researched Cusimano's credentials or specialty, and it seemed like a far-fetched fortuity, but if being my father's doctor once was something that could help my child get closer to a clinic consult with an experienced brain surgeon, I'd use it. Of the few dozen neurosurgeons in the region (they all know each other), what was the chance the one I had a connection to was the one who had experience with this type of tumour?

Dr. Lindgren left me a cellphone message to say he'd faxed a letter to Dr. Cusimano. Hesitating a little just before he signed off, he added, "And ... please call back if you don't get the outcome you want." I didn't know what he meant and couldn't ask a recorded voice. *Call him if we don't go with the other surgeon? Call him if we want to take his team up on their offer to "give it a go" with some scalpels and suction in my son's head? Call him if Cusimano screws up? Call him if our kid doesn't make it? Gets sicker? If we get worse news?* Was medicine a competitive business too? If one salesperson sells you a lemon (even if that lemon is your darling child's future quality of life and the sales dude is a surgeon), then will the next one play the have-I-got-a-deal-for-you game?

It wasn't like I was planning a family vacation and trying to choose between one hotel or another. I didn't want either. I didn't want my son to need a brain surgeon at all. I wanted brain surgeons to go back to being something I joked about not being when I lost my car keys. There was no chance in hell I was going to get the result I wanted, because what I wanted was for it to all disappear. Evaporate. Poof! Like it never happened. I wanted to sweep the reports, test results, and especially diagnostic images under the thickest, heaviest rug I could find. More than anything, I wanted Aaron to go back to being normal in *every* way. I wanted him to forget about the dozen doctors and half as many hospitals. About missing school only to tolerate often rude white-coated strangers standing around him and talking about the size of his hands (Oh my God!), thickness of his tongue (I've never seen anything like it!), or unusual hormonal levels (Did you see the growth hormone this kid has?). I wanted him to knee-jerk respond with his sauciness again when people asked him overly personal questions.

And even though the universe seemed to be intervening, I left nothing to chance. Not anymore. I didn't even wait for the official referral. I located a number for Dr. Cusimano's office and left a long-winded voicemail about whose mother and daughter I was, and the diagnosis we were facing. I wouldn't recommend this approach without the surety I had, having met the doctor and my father being his patient. But the lure of the rare was real too. I had begun to suss out that a rare-disease patient meant access to a rare case, and I could count on that to at least get a reply.

A call the next morning from the surgeon's assistant confirmed Aaron's appointment. I spoke to Samantha in Dr. Cusimano's office at least once a day that month to ensure a complete file was built for Aaron. This was an early lesson that everyone should learn about the medical system — assistants rule. These are the people who control information flow, so make them your best friends. Send them flowers; take them food in their obscurely located, windowless, dull, file-laden offices; introduce them to your adorable child and ask about theirs.

There were hurdles to jump prior to a clinic visit, including a glucose-tolerance test, an MRI, a consult with an endocrinologist, ophthalmic X-rays, and visual-field tests. Samantha scheduled the pre-clinic tests in clusters because we had so far to drive, and she proactively booked pre-surgical admission testing and blood banking with me from the first phone call, anticipating that Dr. Cusimano would take Aaron's case and operate as soon as possible. I thought she was just being efficient and kind. What I should have realized is how at risk my son was. (Yup, we made a personal visit to her office to say thank you and she fist-bumped my kid.) Samantha told me that Dr. Cusimano had done one of these surgeries on a teenager before — after I revealed that I had a few questions ("I'm sorry to bother you, Samantha") because I didn't want to trust what I'd been told by doctors at other hospitals ("I'm sure you can understand I want to be sure").

"It's your son, Mrs. Hall. You ask anything you need to," Samantha reassured me. "Of course you have questions. Yes, he operated on a young man just a few months ago."

"Do you think I could talk to the parents?" I couldn't believe I had the gall to ask. I wanted to talk to someone about pain, risk, and recuperation. About how their child did. I even thought it might be nice for Aaron to know another kid going through this.

I fantasized that the two teenagers might talk about their fears. But I was going to have to get emotionally naked with a stranger, something I had narrowly escaped doing until that point.

Within an hour or two, Samantha got back to me with a man's name and phone number — a local number, in the town next to ours. Another coincidence hit me square in the face. Statistically there could be few teens or children with gigantism in all of Canada. How was it possible that another young man operated on by the same surgeon lived ten minutes from our home? I sat with that phone number for a few minutes. Then I made the call.

"We'd be happy to help, in any way we can," Mike said. He asked about Aaron, but I did most of the talking. Was the surgeon good? Did they know how to handle a kid in that place? How did your son manage? Hormone levels then, and how about now? I learned Brendan had had two operations. But I never asked about his prognosis. Everyone has their own way of coping, of getting their heads around the facts and the risks. I'm a medical-details person. I'd always rather know than not. And at that point, mired in the clinical soup, I was as likely to blurt out that the prognosis was a life expectancy of about twenty-five years old as I was to say the exact name of the tumour or Aaron's growth-hormone level. I had lost my filter. But what worked for me might scare the shit out of people who wanted to know far less. So I had to be careful. I didn't want my research, the fact that I'd dug too deep (maybe), to worsen anything for them. It was all so far over the shock threshold that used to matter in socially appropriate conversation.

"The surgeon was amazing," Mike said. Their son, nineteen years old at the time of my call and completing high school, had procedures six months apart. "The tumour is all gone." Brendan was considered *cured*.

Then it's possible for Aaron too.

"Brendan really needed his mother with him the whole time he was in hospital," Mike said. "It was a scary experience and he didn't want to be alone."

"I expect the same from Aaron." I said that I thought Aaron's surgery would be by the end of the summer, likely August. There was loads of time to prepare. "He's a lovely man, the surgeon," Mike told me. "We really trusted him. More importantly, Brendan trusted him."

These people had done it. Their boy was okay now. This could still just be a horrible few months when Aaron was sixteen and we could look back and be grateful that we'd found the best care for him. I imagined us years ahead, telling the story, made richer by the coincidences that found us a neurosurgeon, of that time when Aaron had a brain tumour.

10

RISK ASSESSOR

I practised how it might go when we met with Dr. Cusimano,
imagining a typical clinic room, the surgeon now in his late
thirties or early forties, the same slender man I'd met across my
father's hospital bed once. I pictured my boy, feet dangling from
the examining-room table, and Rick leaning beside him, arms
folded, ankles crossed. I pre-heard the essential questions. I saw
me managing to stay calm, downplaying the drama, acquiescing
to the demands of my teenager to raise as few issues as possible. I
hoped the doctors wouldn't say too much in front of Aaron, even
though I wanted him to be fully cognizant of what we were discussing and the risks involved. I hoped for his buy-in but I didn't
know what we'd do if he refused to have the operation.

"What if Cusimano won't do it?" Rick had asked me.

"Then we'll go wherever we need to, to find someone
who will." Someone was going to make this go away. Someone,
somewhere.

What do you ask the man who is going to cut into your son's
head? And how do you ask what you really want to know, right

in front of your child? Asking anything the wrong way would get me labelled as *that* mother, a mistake I'd seen my own mother make in so many medical situations, offending by being more aggressive than was warranted, and I wouldn't let my despair take me there. I ran through it in my head instead. I could take the cocky approach, borne of that typical and seemingly ever-present sense of helplessness we all have when dealing with the medical system. I tried out some casual scenarios. "Yeah, so, Doc, how many times have you sliced open someone's nose and pulled out chunks of a tumour? And ... just wondering ... How often does this go very wrong? Oh, and what's the chance my son will die?" *Do I really want to know that?* "And by the way, are you any good at this?" I wondered if I should err on the side of respectful submission, throwing in a little bluntness with some qualifying statement: "Uh, with all due respect" — and much was due — "can you cure my son?" A confident "Of course!" would be nice, please and thank you. Perhaps I would meet him on his own jargon-laced ground: "Dr. Cusimano, how prevalent is the transsphenoidal approach for the resection of a pituitary macroadenoma in your caseload?" I wanted a number. Or I thought I wanted a number, but no number was going to assuage my fears. This was my kid. And what if the information made a decision more difficult? If he said, "Just one," how was I going to feel? Nothing short of a full kid-back guarantee would be good enough. *Good enough.* It was an obscene standard when I considered the measure of success: my son living longer. I wanted more time for Aaron. For us. I needed that doctor, that well-trained man, to buy some time for my kid.

Rick, Aaron, and I sat in another cramped room in another hospital. The lack of space intensified the experience for me — I'd been claustrophobic my entire life. There would be an exam table with the requisite roll of paper attached to the foot, three chairs (at least) and one on wheels, a sink, a blood-pressure meter, and boxes of masks and gloves cluttering a cabinet or desk. The walls bore the connections that I'd seen in so many hospital rooms: a large Emergency button, a red pull-in-case-of-fire switch, an oxygen nozzle. A rolling pole for intravenous bags stood sentry in one corner.

While we waited, Aaron and Rick played with the automatic sink, seeing how quickly they could whip their hands past the sensor without the water turning on, laughing into each other's faces when the other guy's sleeve got wet. It wouldn't be long before they were filling gloves with water and pitching them like water balloons out the windows onto passersby. They played. I stewed.

I wondered how much of this stuff was scripted in medical school. Thinking on their feet in cramped quarters with stressed patients and their families was an occupational reality for surgeons. Was there such a thing as a simple brain-surgery case? One that wasn't urgent? This wasn't a tonsillectomy on a kid who got too many infections. Harried, freaked-out patients were as basic to the work of these doctors as the fluids and tissues they used as markers for illness. The medical profession relies almost entirely on the process of elimination, toward the pursuit of the normal, the average, the baseline range. It isn't this, so it must be that. *Typical* is the place where diagnosticians want to arrive. Aaron was so far outside typical. What happens when they confront the ultra rare and they must surrender themselves to the liminal space where the unknown resides? Wouldn't they all be waffling as much as we were? How do doctors show fear? Would I know it if I saw it?

I sat watching my great-big kid giggling with his father across the room as they nudged each other into filling the first glove. I'd been part of the goofiness on the way there, as the three of us worked the brain-surgeon schtick. Rick came up with, "I wonder if brain surgeons make fun of each other when one of them asks a stupid question, like 'Well, aren't you just a brain surgeon!'"

Dr. Cusimano, a balding, intense, dark-eyed man, entered the examination room as if he was happy to be invited to greet new friends, shaking our hands somewhat more meekly than expected, then formally introducing himself, including title and credentials. His entourage (of only two, I was pleased to see) included the chief neurosurgical resident, a small doctor who focused almost entirely on statistics; and a very young, overly polite medical student who stood behind Dr. Cusimano and nervously adjusted her ponytail and pocket contents. Aaron was seated on an examination table, banging his big black high-cut Nikes against the metal drawers. His little-kid behaviour in a man-sized presence aroused palpable compassion and smiles from all the doctors. I guess it was adorable the first time. I resisted the temptation to tell him to knock it the hell off. It was my hundredth time.

The examination portion took just a few minutes. They measured his head, wrist, and chest using a little blue retractable tape the chief resident produced from his pocket.

"Wow, your wrists are over eight inches around!" the doctor exclaimed.

"Is that good?" Aaron asked, and then offered, "Just wait 'til you measure my fingers!"

"You're not kidding, thirty-three millimetres!" I didn't know if that was big, but I smiled to myself when everyone else in the room held up a hand to compare, wiggling their fingers a little. I noticed Rick's wedding band was gone. Gut punch.

Dr. Cusimano leaned back in an office chair, one ankle crossed over the opposite knee, his fingertips steepled. He wore dark-blue surgical scrubs, and a triangle of curly black hair casually filled the V-neck of his top. He turned to the resident and student next to him.

"What questions would you like to ask Aaron in order to confirm a gigantism diagnosis?" We sat patiently during the teaching moment.

"Headaches, joint pain, vision loss, slowed reflexes, profuse sweating," began the medical student, her words upturned in a question as she spoke.

"Right. Ask the patient," Dr. Cusimano gently directed, and my shoulders relaxed.

Aaron wasn't so polite. In fact, he was tired of having to repeat the details of how sore knees led to mentioning headaches and the CT scan, and that no, he hadn't noticed anything else. So I wasn't surprised when he looked at the doctor and said flatly, "My mom will tell you." I made short work of the highlights, and then Dr. Cusimano began to explain how transsphenoidal surgery would work, advising us what could go wrong while informing us of best outcomes. Aaron kept his face buried in his hands, his head leaned back against the wall, and I caught sight of tears dripping off his chin.

Each piece of carefully delivered science blew me farther and farther off course. I would never be able to find my way back to the fantasy (my delusion) that this wasn't happening. This was brain surgery after all, no matter how much comfort doctors tried to provide by reminding us that they would be in the pituitary cavity or at the base of the brain, not working *on the brain* per se. The brain in question belonged to my boy, so the clinicians could stuff their caveats.

Aaron answered questions about when his headaches began and where in his head they were located, and said yes to every symptom mentioned until the topic came to his stage of puberty, and then he passed the baton back. "Just ask my mom," and the group turned to me.

"Aaron hasn't gone through puberty yet. X-rays showed his bone age is two years younger than his actual age. His testosterone is so low that his growth plates weren't closing as they should have. His pediatric endocrinologist did a complete examination and prescribed testosterone to try to speed things up."

"Has he been prescribed anything else?" Dr. Cusimano asked, pointing to the resident who held the file, which must have been a signal to note down what I said.

"Something for his cortisol, thyroid, and something for his stomach — which is sick a lot. And he'll be starting Sandostatin soon."

Sandostatin was a tumour suppressant, a very expensive drug that had to be given by a nurse or doctor trained to prepare it properly and deliver the injection deep into the hip muscle using a gauge of needle I was certain was meant for an elephant (and later found out it was the largest gauge used on humans), so we would need to travel over an hour for every dose.

"He'll need to stop Sandostatin before surgery," Dr. Cusimano said, "but go ahead and get doses in now. We actually don't know what effect it has on surgical success."

"Should we even start?" I asked.

"That's really up to you." *Thanks for nothing. Up to me.*

"You have a highly operable tumour here. There are risks, extremely rare, but I need to explain them." The list included facial paralysis, pituitary-function worsening, or neurological impairment. I remember hearing about a spinal-fluid leak, meningitis, nasal flow problems, and blood clots. *Do. Not. Look. At. The. Boy.* And then, "There is a risk of death." And just like that the uninvited houseguest was in the room tossing wet towels on the floor again.

Dr. Cusimano gave me a number, a percentage, which I have permanently blocked out because I was squeezing my eyes together, face pointed into my lap, wishing with all my might that Aaron hadn't heard it. The doctor was still talking. "If the carotid artery was nicked and there was bleeding such that we could not control it." He added that MRI reports showed not only that Aaron's tumour was quite large but that it had grown around the carotid. "There is a chance" — he provided another number — "that we would need to open up the cranium because the nasal pathway is not efficient or usable for some reason." In that case Aaron would come out with an incision in his head and staples. Post-op, there could be hormonal imbalances, spinal-fluid leaks, and prolonged bleeding.

I was back at the "risk of death" and pretty sure I'd lost the ability to absorb information after he said it was up to me. But we had to push forward. "What needs to happen before surgery?" I asked.

"Aaron will need to see a neuro-ophthalmologist to assess his pre-surgical optic-nerve status and an ear, nose, and throat surgeon who will do the early and final portion of the procedure." *More specialists ... What the hell is a neuro-ophthalmologist?* Just in that week we had made six trips to the Toronto hospital, three hours in the car each time. He was missing so much school. "And, if you'd like, you can bank your blood here."

There was an awkward moment of silence when I know I simply gazed at Aaron and wondered how he was taking it all in, just hearing that there was a risk he could die or end up paralyzed. I could not believe how calmly the surgeon delivered the details.

Dr. Cusimano explained that if Aaron banked his blood, then if he should need a transfusion he would get his own blood, a choice that increased positive outcomes and lowered risks. I could not even imagine these scenarios.

"At this point are you feeling you would like to proceed, or do you need some time to consider all this?"

Rick and I exchanged glances. I hoped mine said, *Holy fuck, is this guy really asking us to give him permission to cut open our son's head and maybe kill him trying?* It was beyond surreal. This might make me sound like the worst person in the world, but I wished this moment on anyone else.

"What do you think, Aaron?" I asked.

"I say, let's get it over with." He was still teary, his voice crackly.

I turned my face into the wind, found my breath, and said, "What do you need from us?"

II

OATH TAKER

Five adults stood around a room discussing the possibility that a boy could die or need his skull opened or suffer brain damage, paralysis, or other permanent impairments, such as speech difficulties. My sixteen-year-old kid was forced to hear it all, forced to take in information no one should ever have to face, at any age. Instinct told me that the fairest thing to do was to shield him from this, but I didn't know what was fair anymore. Would it be right to just subject him to life-risking surgery without his full awareness? In the eyes of the law, as we were about to learn, his permission was sufficient for treatment. But it seemed unreasonable to me that he consent on his own.

Rick and I were islands, each digesting this information on our own across the room and the gulf that divided us now. We couldn't discuss how we felt, and we couldn't consider alternatives because there weren't any. Going in, we knew that if Dr. Cusimano would take the surgery, we needed to say yes. It was six weeks since diagnosis and fewer since we'd told the kids we were separating, and I so badly wanted to throw myself into Rick's arms and ask for him to carry this, to be the one who walked our boy through the gauntlet. There we stood, ten feet apart, each of us with arms crossed, both biting down hard on our lower lips, wishing beyond everything that we could change the bullshit karma that got us into that room. The separation, the marriage, our failures, and the dissolving of nearly twenty years together didn't matter.

Then it did.

Dr. Cusimano passed papers across the table to us, detailing everything we had been told. I scanned to the bottom of the page, where lines appeared for signatures. My throat tightened. One of the customized points in our custody agreement was my seeking primary medical responsibility for the children. Rick travelled a great deal and I feared finding myself in a situation where I needed to make a judgment call and he was unreachable and couldn't authorize his half of parental responsibilities. Neither of us had a problem with this precaution. But now I saw the metaphorical fine print. Our eyes met as Rick and I both remembered the long-shot situations we'd imagined, which had inspired my insistence upon having clear responsibility, whether he was present or not. I most surely did not want to have primary decision-making responsibility now. Advice to future divorcers: Be careful what you ask for in the settlement.

"I guess you have to sign this," Rick said, and pushed the sheets into my hands, placing the pen on top. Neither of us wanted our freshly inked separation conditions to be outed in that room, so it was a relief when Aaron said, "Why don't we all sign it?" From the mouths of babes.

Rick, Aaron, and I all put our names on that permission form. But I knew the truth: Whatever happened to that boy in surgery was on me. I'd guided him to this point. I'd made the choices. I should have seen it sooner. His life was my job, damn it.

I stole a glance at Aaron. When he met my gaze, I could almost hear him begging me to get him out of there. I knew those eyes — had succumbed to them, read them, and responded to their wordless pleas for sixteen years. I'd always been proud that I could get him the things that he wished for, whatever he needed. I couldn't now, though. I couldn't even come close. I was failing him.

We left feeling some comfort that action was being taken, that we were moving forward. In the car, the three of us agreed that we had confidence in Dr. Cusimano and we felt thankful that, with a proposed surgery date in July, there would be no interruption to the school year.

I guess we thought that mattered still.

Reports from that day reflect how we must have looked to all of them. Our family was well educated on the medical situation, and Dr. Cusimano noted that we were told about risks and our questions were responded to. He ended with what must be a standard remark, that no guarantees were given or implied. And I'd wanted a damned guarantee.

Neuro-ophthalmologists are rare, and Dr. Irene Vanek's time was in great demand. I was told there was not another doctor in the entire metropolitan area around Toronto whose specialty was the diagnosis and treatment of eye tumours. But she squeezed Aaron into her schedule somehow. This woman, who held my teenage son's hand (and he let her) while peering in behind his eyes through machinery that must have cost hundreds of thousands of dollars, saying, "Good boy," and "That's it, my dahlink," and "Just a little longer to be still, my boy," had trained for two decades for the clinical specialty she offered.

We would have travelled hours to see Dr. Vanek again just for her bedside manner, but her impact on Aaron's health journey would ultimately be an equally compelling reason. A five-minute exam involved hearing whether Aaron felt he was having trouble seeing things ("I don't think so") and a couple of minutes in the dark while she shone light through a high-powered microscope to see behind his eyes. "My dahlink boy ... Ve should not vait too long for surgery," she said in her thick Slavik-accented English. And after that one short statement we were out of Dr. Vanek's lovely solar system. I knew from my own reading that without effective treatment to reduce the size of the tumour, it would eventually blind Aaron. I said a silent thank you that she didn't put the word *blind* in the exam room with Aaron present. I could see his sweaty fingerprints on the arms of the chair and wondered if he'd soaked through his shirt during the time in that office.

My questions — "How much time is too long?" and "Should I be asking for an earlier surgery date?" — hung in the air unaddressed, pressed away as she literally shooed us down the hall while handing Aaron a manila file folder to give to a receptionist. "You'll get a call. Bye, bye, dahlink boy." And she left us.

My internet research that night was specifically on risks associated with compression of the optic nerve.

"Do you think they'll hurry up and do my surgery?" he asked. Was that fear or a wish? I was fixated on him finishing his school year. Normalcy. Less lost time. So he wouldn't stand out more than he did. *What are the other kids saying about him already?*

"I'll call Dr. Cusimano's office in a couple of days and make sure he got Dr. Vanek's report about your vision. That's all I can do, I think."

"You could ask them to do it sooner, couldn't you?"

My heart swelled. My son believed that I would be able to do this. He trusted I was on the job, taking care of his medical treatment. Maybe he didn't blame me. "I can try, Aaron. But you'll miss school, buddy."

He was quiet for a moment, busy ploughing through a fat corned-beef sandwich, bag of chips, and two massive cookies he had insisted on getting from the Shopsy's across from the hospital. The habit of feeding him after appointments, when the anxiety had abated and the butterflies in his stomach quieted into a hunger he was not willing to let me ignore, kept him quietly feasting for the first twenty minutes of our long highway drive home.

"I don't care anymore, Mom."

"About what?" I didn't know if he was about to be profound or mouth off with some prickish teenager remark.

"I don't care about missing school, waiting 'til after June." He chewed. "I don't care about anything anymore." And then the fear broke through. "Am I going blind, Mom?"

Fuck. That hadn't been on my radar. I didn't have the answer. Wasn't it bad enough that the kid's looks were changing? He was taller than 99 percent of the Canadian (and likely the world's) population; he walked in pain; he couldn't take a long adulthood for granted, like other entitled teens; and now the spectre of blindness was added to the mix.

"I wish I knew the answer, Aaron. But I'll get you one."

"What if I wake up tomorrow and I can't see? What if the tumour moves or something?"

He was right, maybe. I supposed anything like that was possible, but I tried to tell him what my rational mind decided. "I think that if going blind really quickly was possible, you would be in surgery right now. I don't think that brilliant woman would have let us leave if there was chance you would go blind before the surgeons get you a date."

But everything I was saying was bullshit. I had no idea.

On the phone, where the boys couldn't hear us, Rick and I went over the logistics. We were handling things from two houses now. The movers had come, emptied my stuff out of the garage, and were transferring a couple of pieces of furniture (my family antiques, my piano, and things that Rick had built for me) to the house I'd purchased in town. It was a blur, and the unpacking was such a low priority that I did it only when the boys were not at home. Salt in the wound, if they were watching.

In our usual style Rick and I split the tasks we could, making lists, our shared forte. Rick had worked a minimum ten-hour day, at least five days a week, his entire working life. He was a steadily climbing executive in an auto-parts-manufacturing operation with three factories in southern Ontario. He left appointments to me because his schedule limited his availability and that was how he had always done things. He would drive Aaron and Justin wherever they needed to go on weekends and attend appointments if I asked him to, but there was very little he could do during the week. It had always been this way and after Aaron's diagnosis; he expected I would just take on the extra, and I did.

I booked meetings with Aaron's vice-principal and guidance counsellor, as well as with Justin's teacher, because I had a suspicion that if it hadn't already, their school performance was likely to be affected by the stress around our house, and their behaviour might be also.

I felt compelled to hurry, to make things happen as quickly as I could. Because, well, his life depended on it. These months before his surgery imbued my daily life, my waking hours, with a sense of urgency so profound, its anxiety-provoking tentacles are still my constant companions.

If the gap between appointments, procedures, or tests stretched too long, it meant time wasted and more growth for Aaron — and the earlier onset of symptoms. Every inch of height put pressure on his organs, bones, and spine, which would expedite the crippling pain that I had learned all giants lived with. And the taller he got, the more he would stand out. And that meant more stigma and more derision. I so badly wanted my boy to escape both the symptoms *and* the mistreatment. But even if I could only minimize his symptoms, I was going to rush like a mad fool.

In the car one day, not two weeks after we saw Dr. Vanek, Aaron said, "I can't see your hands in the car anymore."

"Whaddya mean?" I said, thinking he was being funny. "My hands are right here, on the steering wheel."

"I'm serious, Mom. When I'm looking out the front window and you're talking, like y'always do, with your hands" — he stopped to imitate me, contorting his hands into mock sprinklers spurting invisible confetti — "I don't see them moving, anymore."

In my mind, I heard his question again: *Am I going blind, Mom?*

A band of panic tightened across my middle. *Has he been losing his sight all this time and not bothered to say anything? Or has he been ignoring it? Did we both miss this?* "How long has it been like this?"

"I just noticed. I think."

Face palm. Now was not the time to point out that he might have told Dr. Vanek this nor to jab him with "you really shoulda told me, son," because above all, I needed Aaron to keep talking, to keep telling me *everything*. For all I knew there would be other symptoms I couldn't predict, and his telling me would be the only warning. His trust in me and his talkativeness were our early warning system, our DEW Line. His health outcome and maybe our relationship's survival depended on me managing my reaction: not too Mom, not too buddy. He was a teenage boy, after all, who had no reason to want to share a damn thing with his mom. I made a mental note: Do whatever it takes to be the person he *always* wants to talk to and spend time with. I had to stack the deck in his favour, and I'd swallow my tongue to do it.

12

NURSE

We had a comfortable two months before surgery. I had a dedicated notebook, and I'd made checklists, putting the essential dates on the family calendar on the fridge, so the boys would be prepared for what was coming. They would finish their year at school, and Reef's training would be wrapped up for the semester. By June we'd be more settled in the new house. I'd get the boys' rooms decorated as they wanted (dark primary colours, even at their ages) and I could get some flower beds planted. Plenty of time to organize how I could be with Aaron at the hospital for his surgery days and arrange day camps for Justin.

So when I answered the phone on April 30 and Dr. Cusimano's assistant asked me if I could manage if Aaron was admitted five days from now, I was so surprised I asked, "For what?" Already accustomed to my sense of humour, she paused and then told me that Aaron's procedure had been moved up to the first date available on the surgical roster. I didn't need to ask why. You don't get moved up this kind of roster just because you're a sweet kid. Dr. Vanek's report advised that he needed surgery right away because the tumour was compromising the optic nerve and the damage could be irreversible. What Aaron noticed in the car *was* happening. The same way he'd thought something was in his head. The first wave of artillery had come over the knoll.

And just as he became an emergency, I became his first responder. Barking orders and marshalling coverage. I called Rick. He'd need to be off work. Then I scanned my mental horizon for my next move. I called Val. I couldn't risk overthinking this. She'd steady me. "We don't have any more time," I blurted when she answered.

"What? Has something happened since I talked to you yesterday? Is Aaron okay?" she asked.

I hadn't seen my girlfriends much. I'd lost track of how long it had been since I met Val or Dana for a cup of coffee. I'd lost track of most things. I was too preoccupied scanning the waters ahead for potential menaces to bother eating (I hardly did), seeking support (I didn't), or considering self-care (never, nothing, nada).

"I'll help," Val said. "Just do what you need to for Aaron and give me a list." There she was, willing to do anything, everything, and I'd been missing her calls and not responding to her messages for weeks.

Twenty minutes later, I had a new plan. Rick and I would take him in together. One of us expected to sleep at the hospital and the other would be with Justin. I packed a bag to move to the hospital for the duration if needed. Val moved in with us at my new house, offering to help with dogs, errands, driving, whatever. I had a massive master bedroom, so we added her queen-sized bed to it. I had no idea what would happen or what Aaron would need. I admit to myself now that I didn't even know if I'd have Aaron.

Val was fourteen years younger than me, and just a teenager when her mother, a neighbour, volunteered to work with me in Kiddo Knits, a children's knitwear-design company I was running, mostly to stay sane while my kids were preschoolers. Her mother could knit anything I dreamed up, from three-dimensional chenille flowers to hats that made babies looks like heads of cabbage. In an effort to get me more time for designing and later, to write, Val became an afterschool babysitter. She was mature beyond her years and reminded me of myself when I was a fish out of water in high school: enamoured of the world of literature, dogged by the tiresome bullshit of teenage girls. Val adored my kids and seemed to get me and my firm pick-my-battles parenting style. The "getting me" never ended. I was mentor to her and she was the little sister I'd never had, without the complications of blood relations and implied responsibilities. She was my best friend before I knew it, my substitute, intuitively able to suss out what I would want done for a wailing preschooler with a grazed knee and independently tasking herself with taking my car, my kids, and my Visa and doing the grocery shopping. When the boys were old enough to no longer need a caregiver, she had an organic role with us that defied a label. She was my go-to, the boys' backup parent, and they had complete comfort with her and trust that she would both be their buddy and enforce Mom and Dad's rules. So when my coping skills withered and shame grew as I realized I needed to leave my marriage, she was devastated. She felt she'd have to choose Rick or me. She couldn't be split down the middle. She chose me. I needed her but I felt like I'd ripped her off too.

I had no idea what extent she would go to in order to save me from myself but I soon learned. I was slipping up on a lot of things, not just because I was spending the bulk of my days driving Aaron to appointments, but also because I was losing my focus like someone night marched at gunpoint. In the lead up to this, in the aftermath of moving to my own house, a lot of things had to go. Yoga classes, writing group, volunteering on a charity board, and heartbreakingly, Reef.

The requirements for raising Reef involved both maintaining his training regimen at home and taking him to the training facility three mornings a week. I would need to be gone for at least five days after Aaron's surgery, and even longer if something unforeseen kept Aaron admitted; we were already having difficulty keeping up with our commitment to the charity and to the caramel-coloured golden retriever whose training Aaron felt strongly about participating in. Reef needed to go live with someone else.

Two days after the new surgery date was dropped on me, I dropped a bomb of my own — "Reefy needs to go back, buddy." Aaron and I were outside together practising Reef's recall in an exercise we enjoyed called Puppy Ping-Pong. Aaron and I alternately called Reef to us from increasing distances apart, strengthening his ability to stay focused on the verbal command for when, in public demonstrations, people nearby clapped and tried to distract him.

Aaron frowned at me. "Whaddya mean, back?"

"To the charity," I said. "We can't look after him the way we're supposed to, and … we won't be here for at least a week, and … we don't know about after …"

"You can't take Reef from me too, Mom." Aaron squatted and pulled Reef into his chest. Reef obliged and licked his face.

"He isn't ours, buddy. You know he'll leave us permanently one day to go into service. We have to think of his training. We aren't here enough, and we'll be away."

"You're freaking kidding me? You're gonna take my best friend away, right when I'm goin' in the hospital to have my head cut open?" Shoulders pulled up around his ears, chest puffed out. Aaron threw the red training toy as hard as he could against the backyard fence and whipped open the sliding-glass door. Reef bounded after him, likewise turning his back on me and holding me responsible for this unthinkable slag.

"I'm going with Reef now, Aaron," I called up the stairs the next afternoon.

"I'm not coming down, Mom. I can't see him again."

The owner of the charity would keep Reef at her own home until a replacement family was found for him. It wasn't fair to send him to another home and then to ask for him back when it was more convenient for us; we'd have to forfeit the remaining months of training time with him. I rationalized that Reef was almost two and would be tested and pass into some kind of service role in a few months anyway. I also hoped that in this confusing and stressful time, the ache at Reef being gone from our lives would be eased. We had two other dogs, Spirit and Maddie, and with the addition of Val's massive Bernese mountain dog, Layla, our house was overflowing to the point of bedlam. Would all the chaos mask yet another loss?

Luckily we'd already completed pre-op. So it wasn't part of what we had to mash into that five-day window. A week or so before Samantha's call to move up the surgery, we'd sat in a closet-sized exam room across from a little desk with a tent card on it that read "Pre-Op Clinic." A rushed but kind nurse went down a checklist of tests completed, mentioned that we should bring pyjamas but warned not to bring anything else because "things do get stolen around here." Aaron was eating the last of a Nutri-Grain bar when a good-looking man sporting crisply pressed scrubs came into the room with a clipboard. He was in his forties with dark well-styled hair and black hipster glasses, and he went directly to shake Aaron's hand. No remarks about Aaron's size, his hands, anything. He had me at the handshake. The nurse excused herself. She had a good scoop to go tell in the coffee room now about the giant kid.

Dr. Penoit took a medical history and explained how the surgery day was going to work. He discussed a rare blood condition in our family, one that Rick had been troubled by, having been hospitalized for two blood clots. This sticky-blood factor increased the risk of clotting, and therefore, of aneurysm. He circled something on the clipboard sheets, said we'd be seeing a hematologist (*There's a new one*), and he would have to bring this up with the surgical team. He learned we had a family history of heart problems, a case of flesh-eating disease, childhood kidney diseases, cancer, rheumatic fever, and geriatric diabetes. Aaron was fit for surgery, but his anxiety was noted, and the attentive physician prescribed Ativan for the operating room, stating (quite warmly, I thought, when I read his notes later) that Aaron "wants to remember as little as possible of the OR experience."

On the drive home Aaron reminded me how much he hated having his blood taken: "Remember — banking my blood was the worst experience yet." He'd nearly squeezed my hands to the point of broken bones. I didn't need reminding.

Back in the car after our long day at the hospital, in a gap between Aaron's complaints — I wanted so badly to tune him out but feared I'd miss something important — Aaron said something so quietly, I barely heard him. "Every time I close my eyes I picture myself on the operating table completely out of control." He told me that in this vision or dream or nightmare, he was pinned down and that scared him most of all. He didn't want to be asleep and splayed open on the table. "Like on television," he said.

"Those are autopsies, bud, and they weren't real." The point was lost on him. Fear had the helm. Every fiction had some fact in it, now, thanks to the terror. I wished I'd never exposed my kids to media at all. I should've given more thought to raising them off grid in the Himalayas.

"But they can't do anything about it." He couldn't do anything about this. My heart was broken.

I thought about my own history. Post-op pain was what I would have feared in his place. But he had no point of reference. He had never known the bleariness of coming out of anesthetic. He had no experience with pain or pain killers for that matter. He had not been through hospital nights when a nurse awakens you every couple of hours and the annoyance of beeping monitors and pump alarms. But he knew what helplessness felt like, so he went there.

His relative innocence was shattered. Boyhood was over. His privacy threatened, his self-image now so difficult to nurture, he would be drawn into a place between childhood and adulthood without a firm sense of belonging to either.

"Mom?" he asked, after being asleep for part of the trip.

"Yeah, bud?"

"There's a good chance I won't survive this, isn't there?" *Does he mean surgery, the disease, the tumour, what?*

"I can't believe you won't, Aaron. I won't believe that. You can't either."

On the day before Aaron's admission to hospital, as I drove Justin home from school, his questions from the back seat should have struck me as too off the cuff and calm, but in my fogginess I just answered them as they came.

"So, tomorrow I might not have a brother anymore?" Justin was brave enough to ask what I could not allow myself to think.

"You mean if he doesn't survive the surgery," I said, not really asking. My voice was flat, monotone, like the asphalt view through my windshield.

"Yeah. He could die in brain surgery, right?"

"Yes, he could. Anyone could die in any surgery, I guess. But Aaron's surgery is really close to his brain and the big arteries that feed it with blood."

"Tonight might be the last time I see him, then," he said.

I felt like I had bitten off my tongue. I hadn't known how Justin was feeling about everything, because I hadn't wanted to push a conversation on him. We didn't have that kind of time anymore. I hated myself for not being as present for Justin these last few months. Both boys were still adjusting to the two-house schedule of being at Dad's some nights and Mom's new home all the rest. He'd been coping with his parents breaking up. I'd been keeping my head under the proverbial blankets, denying anything else mattered but Aaron's medical diagnosis. I didn't want to hear about the impact of the move, the separation, this time, what I'd done. I'd failed Aaron by not seeing his illness, not getting on it faster, and that was epic. I couldn't face wrecking Justin's life and Rick's too.

In an email to a bunch of friends with my new address and landline number, I managed my on-stage Patti effervescence for public consumption. "Justin has a new fish named Tyrone. My cellphone is the same and I never will be again." The truth was that I was floundering; I didn't know how be in the *normal* mothering place with one child and in the *sick kid* mothering place with another, at the same time.

I hope Justin never holds me accountable for how badly I ripped him off in those months, and maybe even sometimes in the years that followed, because I surely did. The rushed bedtimes. Not dropping into school anymore or going on field trips as the cool chaperone parent. Fewer of those surprise burger lunches, and a lot more "I don't have time," "I'm sorry," and "maybe later," which ultimately turned into "Sorry, Jay, I just can't do it" or more often still, me whispering, "I love you more than anything" through my sobs from his bedroom door, to what I could see of the profile of his face where he'd fallen asleep waiting on me. Failing Justin may have hurt most of all.

The surgery was scheduled on the same day that Justin's Grade 8 graduation photos were being taken. The humour wasn't lost on us, sandwiched between the horrible and the ridiculous. Rick and I snickered on a phone call, each of us trying to one-up the other as we planned the logistics of the morning.

"While Aaron's having brain surgery, let's put every effort into the shit that *truly* matters and ensure Justin has a crisp white shirt and his curls are perfect," Rick said.

"Oh yeah, and while we're pacing the hospital hallways, waiting to hear if Aaron has survived, let's put our copious amount of spare energy into worrying Justin has matching socks," I added. You don't choose the way endurance comes; you just jump on the bandwagon.

At 4:00 a.m. three of us set off for St. Michael's Hospital in Toronto. Aaron leaned forward over the console between the front seats where Rick and I sat, as if we were off on an exciting road trip instead of to the hospital for a life-threatening operation. He talked nonstop, question after question about detail after detail, his anxiety driving him toward everything we could possibly tell him that might prepare him more for this gargantuan unknown. Our usual routine for any road trip was to get coffee, drinks, and bagels with cream cheese along the way, and the shock of not making our regular stops punctuated the atmosphere in the car. I felt like I had to point out the obvious. "We won't eat, buddy, because you're fasting and that would be cruel."

"I don't care," he said, "it's not like I'd touch a coffee if you paid me. Well, maybe, for the right amount of cash." He snickered. "I just want to not have to think about it. I want to get there and be asleep and know nothing and be done." He fidgeted in his seat, propped his head on a pillow against the window, and kept the questions coming. Had I remembered to pack his toothbrush and toothpaste? Where would his pyjamas be after surgery? Would he have his underwear on? Would his head be wrapped in bandages? What about his iPod?

I tried to sound blasé. "It's in my bag, Aaron. Everything is in my bag."

"I know. I just keep tryin' to think of everything that might go wrong. So I don't think about what's gonna happen, because no one can tell me what *is* gonna happen."

"Well, if your iPod and toothbrush are at the top of the worry list, I think you're doing great, pal," Rick chimed in, making us laugh.

"It's better than thinkin' about a bunch of doctors standin' around me while they put me to sleep and cut into my head."

That statement hung in the air while we all drowned in the image.

"You won't know what's happening, sweetie, because you'll be asleep, remember? I promise." Did my voice sound as soothing as I hoped?

"Is there a chance I could wake up in the middle? I've thought about that, dreamed about wakin' up with masked strangers around me and I'm stuck there on the table, being held down even, by straps or something."

"No, there is no chance," I said. "You'll meet the anesthesiologist, the doctor whose one job it is to keep you under at exactly the right level for exactly as long as Dr. Cusimano needs. The anesthesiologist never leaves your side."

I watched the landscape whip by in the early morning. Surreal in the grey-blue near dawn. I fought to stay in the car, glanced at the door handle. I wanted to be what he needed, seem not fearful, but I also wanted to do a movie stuntwoman roll from the car and not survive it.

"I just don't want to know it's happening." He was asking, not telling.

My heart was aching. "You won't. I promise you won't." Another promise I made, knowing I had no control over its keeping.

Then another set of questions. "How will I feel when I wake up?"

I hadn't considered post-op to that point. "I'm sure your head will ache. You might feel sick to your stomach because of the anesthetic. Your nose will have bandages and maybe gauze inside. There will be a nurse with you all the time in the recovery area. They might ask you if you feel like you're going to throw up. If you need to, make sure you tell them. If you feel pain, then be honest about it."

"Will you be there when I wake up?"

"I'll get to you as soon as I can. As soon as they let me. I promise. You'll be sleepy and feel groggy, so you won't be noticing how much time has passed or whether I'm there yet or not."

Inside the waiting room for surgical patients were persons at every age, every stage of life and physical ability. My son was clearly the youngest, and as always, the largest. He looked too healthy to be going into surgery.

A nurse roaming with a clipboard checked off patients seated on gurneys, put hospital bracelets on them and then cross-referenced the information on the bracelets with what people told her about their name and date of birth, then placed their hands back in their laps. Orderlies wheeled bed after bed through double doors at the far end of the brightly lit room. I was having creepy visions of internment camps.

"Mom, why's your face so red?" Aaron asked. My strain was showing.

"What?" I lifted my hands to my cheeks and raised my eyebrows in a question to Rick.

Aaron wore a blue hospital gown, his black-socked feet hung out over the end of the gurney, comically huge and dark in a place of crisp whites, hospital greens, and sanitizing blues. I'd covered him with two flannel blankets, fresh from the warmer. Aaron never felt the cold, but it comforted me to give the blankets to him. It was something I could do. Aaron leaned back against Rick, who had his arms around our boy's shoulders, their two pairs of huge hands wrapped in one another's. My child's face, his father's chocolate-drop eyes, my dad's curly hair, the profile of the infant on the ultrasound. I was wavering on my feet, steadying my shaking by touching my fingertips to the bed's end. I was dissolving. I couldn't lose it here in front of him. I watched the clock. I tried looking around the pre-op ward and only reassured myself that yes, I was the most terrified-looking person there. The risks ran through my head, his blood factor, the history of heart problems in my family, his carotid artery encased in tumour, and we didn't know how he would do under anesthetic.

Four people in scrubs stepped through the grey swinging doors and walked toward us: the neurosurgeon, an anesthesiologist, and two ENTs (ear, nose, and throat surgeons). The consult was over in minutes, and then Aaron was on the surgical bed, the warmed flannel blankets pulled up to his chest, big round eyes slippery with tears, being pulled away from where we stood. He kept eye contact, turning his head awkwardly over his shoulder, until he was swallowed up by the hallway beyond the doors.

He was at once and again the infant peering at me over the shoulder of the nurse, after a night of being forcibly fasted, going into a place where I could not protect him, where I'd authorized sending him. *What kind of monster was I?*

How do I say goodbye? How could I say I love you enough to comfort him for the moment and myself for forever? The wailing, pleading mantra from within me was there again.

Please, not my baby … Please, not my baby …

I have no idea if we said goodbye.

He bravely went in, nearly on time, I texted my sister. And she emailed exactly that to twenty or so of my friends and family.

We had been through health crises when Aaron was an infant. But the fifteen years in between had left me out of practice, and I admit that we took the boys' amazing health, strong personalities, and wonderful brains for granted. I scolded myself often for that.

I'd spent the month before Aaron was born in the hospital with toxemia. A few days before his premature birth, I'd been allowed to go home for the weekend, since there was no indication of the baby having engaged (moved toward or into the birth canal) or being in trouble. But there had to be a nurse with me to check my blood pressure and heart rate every two hours, including in the night. My mother made it possible for me to be home doing nesting tasks like folding baby blankets and baking muffins on the morning labour gripped me in its vice. When I called the hospital, the responding nurse was very concerned that I hurry in immediately. She must have pulled my chart.

It was a high-risk labour; I was sure I heard the sound of a helicopter's rotors spinning above us on the maternity ward roof accompanying my contractions. After nearly every intervention possible, including vacuum extraction and clipping an electrode to his scalp to monitor his heart rate, Aaron was born into an obstetrician's hands and immediately transferred to Dr. Tobin for the APGAR examination. I remember her handing the baby to Rick after doing the check and saying, "He is perfect."

Dr. Tobin was as composed standing nearby during that stressful labour as she was there beside my tearful teenager in February 2009. His surprise early birth was only a preview of the crises that dotted our first year together. I remembered how Rick managed back then, guided by the resolute demeanour of Dr. Tobin, and I hoped I could use her calmness as an inspiration again. I had wanted to ask if it all seemed as bizarre to her as it did to me that day in the office when we spoke discreetly about symptoms, both sensing the other knew where the examination was heading; that this almost-man, twice her size, was the same child who was born so tiny, although larger than the pre-birth ultrasound predicted, at five pounds thirteen ounces, in crisis then and in crisis now in his teens.

Aaron was severely jaundiced and did not nurse well in the beginning, largely due to interruptions to spend time under blue lights in an isolette in Neonatal Intensive Care until his jaundice level peaked. As is often the case, time away from me did not encourage his latch or our bond. Even after many days at home, his eyes were yellow and his skin had an orangey tone, and his feeding challenges continued. Aaron did not gain weight significantly for two weeks, dropping below five pounds, a situation that combined with the jaundice and feeding problem became very concerning to a diligent Dr. Tobin, who we visited every other day in those first weeks.

During one of those regular visits, she palpated his scalp where the fetal electrode had been clipped and noticed a pocket of trapped fluid on the top of Aaron's head, about the diameter of a golf ball. The first crisis was upon us and he was not even five pounds. I couldn't believe I hadn't felt it, but baby Aaron had worn little hand-knit caps about the size of my palm from the second he was born. The hospital staff put a pale-blue preemie cap on him when his tiny head was wiped clean, and a gentle nurse tucked him, swaddled, under the warming lights. I kept a cap on him even when I bathed him so he would not lose body heat. I felt like the worst new mother ever, not seeing such a large flaw on my perfect little guy's body, and there I was handling him constantly.

At eight weeks old, the second crisis hit. An abdominal hernia erupted when we were in Dr. Tobin's office for a yet another routine weigh-in. She was placid under stress while my baby screamed on my shoulder that day. More high-pitched screams burst out of him the moment I laid him down to diaper him in the exam room. Dr. Tobin had stepped out to take a phone call. She came running back instantly when the new strength of wailing began. It was not a hungry, wet, or tired cry — it was pain. He was nearly blue with the effort to be heard. "Let me," Dr. Tobin said and she peeled open his diaper. I thought maybe a tab was poking him or he had a burning rash. I saw a large fleshy lump about half the length of my thumb protruding to the right of his belly button. She simply pressed it back into his body. It was as if his muscles had split open underneath and his innards were coming out. I was horrified that it was happening to my baby. It was surreal. I bent from the waist and put my forearms on the exam table, leaning in to press little kisses on my wailing baby's fleshy cheek and to quell the rising of whatever my panic attack was forcing up into my throat while she wrapped Aaron tightly in his flannel receiving blanket — I remember it was the one I sewed myself, with little lions on it — and said, "I already called the hospital. Go straight to emerg. Don't even park. They're expecting you. Hurry."

I hustled to the door with Aaron buckled in his baby seat over my one arm, and grabbed the diaper bag from the floor beside my wide-eyed mother.

"It will need to be surgically repaired," Dr. Tobin said, reaching to hold the office door open for us. "I'll call you at the hospital in an hour."

I can't remember the faces of the mothers who must have heard the screams and saw the flurry of activity around that examining room. I don't recall getting to the car. I guess my mother followed along after me.

My mother sat in the back with Aaron, and I told her to take him out of the car seat and hold him, laws and risk be damned. I couldn't bear to let him cry, and I didn't know how serious the rupture could get if he continued to scream. I raced a few blocks to the hospital. In my rear-view mirror, my mom held him tight to her chest, tears streaming down her face, rubbing her damp cheek against his.

They repaired the hernia a few weeks later, surgery that required special permissions from the provincial ministry to be performed on a child so young, in a regional hospital. After the procedure, three nurses (two pushing poles with lines running from them into my boy's tiny body) rushed to get him into my arms, knowing what we both needed, me and my breastfed infant, who had been held nearly every moment since I'd brought him home until I handed him to medical strangers that morning. I peeled open whatever I was wearing, hiked up my breastfeeding T-shirt and got my tiny boy, all tubes and tape and electrodes, next to my bare chest, and I curled around him and wailed. They stood back and let me. I felt observed, like a museum exhibit under glass, but my body and soul were consumed by the sympathy I had for that little person. I belonged to him. My body, my heart, my life belonged to him then, if not before. I was born to be this child's mother.

I felt responsible for getting him to the pain and equally responsible to get him out of it. We were prisoners together, bound by my anguish and my commitment to mothering him.

13

SENTRY

Not knowing what the day would be like, how we would hold our emotions together, what Aaron would look like or feel like after the transsphenoidal surgery, or what calls to action the aftermath might require, I forced my attention onto the minutiae I could control. I went sock shopping. I didn't want to overinflate the importance of what I was doing. I knew I would always remember what I'd bought that day and thought perhaps I should purchase something significant. Like art? A car? Something for Aaron? But then, what if things went horribly wrong? What would anything matter?

I didn't need socks. And in early May, I wouldn't be wearing them. I bought six pairs of bright royal-blue socks — the colour people who know me call "Patti-blue" — and two pairs of shoes and then I dragged a full knapsack and shopping bags for blocks across two downtown university districts. If it had been later in the day, I might have holed up with my notebook in a pub.

I was a boiling cauldron, grateful to the unknowing passersby who gave me fodder for resentment. I feel a little ashamed now of how I was hating on every person whose life was still going on unabated, untouched by the horror my son was enduring as instruments bored into his head, but it made the time easier to bide. Like I said, I'm ashamed now. I walked by self-absorbed students with phones in one hand and lattes from Starbucks in the other. People just kept on hurrying to the places they told themselves mattered. I was a curled lip, snarling dog, glaring at them all in their busyness, hurling whispered obscenities under my breath. I wanted the world to stop turning, to halt mid-stride and hold its collective breath until my son came out alive. My boy was on a surgeon's table, and why did the world not get that?

Rick preferred being productive and *doing*; he needed a task for distraction. While I preferred to stay nearby the hospital and endure the waiting. He drove the hour north of Toronto to pick Justin up from school. We'd been told to expect it would be many hours before we could see Aaron. I texted updates to my sister, Kelly, so I could avoid answering queries from too many people, then resumed walking the city, storm cloud over my head and an anvil on my shoulders. Rick and I had agreed that no family members should come because our families had never interacted comfortably, and we didn't need to be refereeing that day. We didn't know what we'd be in for and having an audience was not something we could stand if we were going to fall apart.

I hadn't wanted anyone in the family, not even Val or Dana, to be with me that day. I knew I'd have no emotional bandwidth to attend to someone's questions, listen to their small talk, or be concerned if I was being polite. I couldn't be a good friend on a day when I didn't even know how to be comforted by one. But Nancy, the unstoppable ball-of-energy mom to Brendan, the other young man with gigantism who shared Aaron's surgeon, would not take no for an answer. She came by bus to meet me. I remember her saying she came because "she couldn't believe I was all alone doing this." I warmed to her candour. She walked into the famous downtown restaurant where, on my tenth cup of coffee, I sat journalling and studying the storied face of Massey Hall. My feet weren't touching the ground and I wasn't in my body. She was kind and chatty and forthcoming with memories of when Brendan had his surgeries a year or more before. I don't know if I chatted, ignored her, or stared into the distance. I may have shared my deepest secrets. I likely tried to eat. And she is a mom, so she undoubtedly got me to eat something. We may have walked. We might have run naked through Dundas Square. I've been too afraid to ask her about those hours in the years that have ensued.

At some point I found myself with a massive coffee in one hand, wedged into a chair in the busy lobby of the hospital with my bags and knapsack and notebook, making pack-mule references about myself. Nancy must have been nearby; she probably bought the coffee and was pouring it into me too. Aaron had been in the operating room for six hours by then. There was nowhere to wait except in this most public of places, a suffocating thoroughfare of a space adapted from the original heritage building and retrofitted to serve as both vestibule and way-finding stop-off, with its floor-to-ceiling wall-mounted boards with clinic names, arrows, and floor numbers. There were always a couple of people craning their necks up to read the wall (Didn't anybody think about how difficult these things are to read?) and hundreds streamed by from various wings of the cobbled-together edifice. It was a claustrophobe's nightmare.

My mind was ablaze, running scenarios. *Shouldn't I have heard something by now? Did my phone battery die? Why haven't they called me yet? Is it better to hear something, or is this a no-news-is-good-news kinda thing?* I felt certain by then that if something horrific had occurred, my phone would have rung. Sitting still was risky. Time to think was a chasm drop, when fears — rational and ludicrous — could consume me, and I'd avoided crashing into a meltdown so far. I could hear my panting breath inside my head, feel the heat in my face, and I tried to people-watch with a fierce, sweaty grip on my cellphone. I raised my eyes from it and there he was — Archangel Michael. A marble sculpture of him stood just a few feet away.

How did I not see him before? I'd walked through this lobby a dozen times. He was captivating, arresting, personable yet impossibly beautiful. There was no way to interpret this sculpture as an *it*, the work was a *he*. Eyes downcast to his left, perhaps resting on the tip of his sword below, he was armoured, winged, and caped. This Michael was the epitome of the graceful strength I wished I had. A brochure nearby informed me that the angel was the symbol of the hospital, offering hope and healing to people of many faiths. The hospital would later call itself the Urban Angel in marketing campaigns, emblazoning Michael across blue-toned posters on the building facades.

I looked at him intently.

Where was my faith? Would better mothers be praying now, huddled in the shadows of the hospital chapel, crouched on bent knees, begging for mercy or sequestered in a pew whispering pleas in the landmark cathedral a block away? I'd known powerful experiences of faith in my life, including the warm feeling of assurance I carried with me at summer bible camp when I was ten and my counsellor Tinker told me that was what God felt like, but now I sensed only the despair of being at the mercy of humans, however well-intentioned and trained. I wanted it not to be true, that only humans could save my boy now. I wanted a cavalcade of angels but I didn't deserve them. Isn't that how faith works? Does God only show up for the loyal, the praying, the church attendees? My boy deserved an angel and my failure as a Christian shouldn't rob him of that. But I felt that it did.

The hospital flyer told the story of nuns who had found the marble sculpture blackened and forgotten in a second-hand shop, and purchased it for forty-nine dollars over a hundred years ago. Recently, a scratching on the back was discovered that confirmed the marble source was the same as that of Michelangelo's work. A great story, a breathtaking piece of art, but it did not bring me comfort, because I wondered where the hell the God I thought I knew was when he let children be stricken with crippling ailments, diseases with unknown origins, and pitiful prognoses. Instead of a prayer, I offered an embittered rant, a rail against a God whose motives I shamefully, selfishly queried. Even after surgery, if — rather, *when* he survived — Aaron's life could be cut drastically short, he could be physically and painfully disabled, and I'd read about how he could require a lifetime of cancer-causing, expensive medication, radiation treatments, specialists, medication supports, therapists, and who knows what else?

He might never have children and could suffer bone-bending deformities in his limbs. And then there was the stigma, that pointing, questioning, indiscreet, sneaky phone photo-taking. Where was God now? Where was Archangel Michael, the protector of children, when my boy needed him? I needed an angel. What would Rabbi Harold Kushner tell me? He wrote his famous book, *When Bad Things Happen to Good People*, some years after his son, also named Aaron, died at fourteen due to progeria. Kushner worked out where God had been for him, reconciling the unfathomable — the loss of his child. I needed the Rabbi's lucidity now.

My inner plea, so loud I could hear nothing else, suppressed my rant. *Please, not my baby … Please, not my baby …* Usually it repeated on an endless loop but music stopped it this time. A choir in fact, but not the heavenly host. A group of children in white shirts were singing Alabama's "Angels Among Us." *Isn't that about a mother who can't see an angel?*

Rick called to say he and Justin were on their way to the hospital. I checked in at the surgical reception desk, where a young man handed me a folded slip of paper: Aaron will be in NICU, M.C.

Michael Cusimano. It was after 3:00 p.m. After seven hours, Aaron's surgery was complete.

I couldn't remember a time I hadn't known where my kid was or what was happening to him for seven hours. I swam in the warm bathwater of relief. Nancy and I headed straight up to the Neurosurgical Intensive Care Unit. Our tone had lightened, and I made fun of how out of shape all this stress was making me feel as we tromped up the flights of stairs and down the hall, and I was short of breath. Maybe I'd been holding my breath. Nancy stood beside me as I lifted the receiver off its cradle on the wall, which automatically rings the busy nurses' station. A moment later, I blurted, "What do you mean he isn't there?" Nancy grabbed my elbow and I turned to her. "Where is he?"

"We need to go to the OR," Nancy said.

"We can't just go walking into the OR, for God's sake."

"We sure as heck can," she said. "They've lost your boy."

We turned for the elevator and bumped squarely into the anesthesiologist we had met that morning in the waiting area. My stricken expression was a giveaway.

Skipping uncalled-for pleasantries, which no clinician really has the skills for at any time, he said, "Your boy did really well. Have you seen him?"

"We can't find him," I said.

The tears took over then, and thankfully, so did Nancy's more-practised-than-mine Grizzly Mom, right up to the operating-room doors and right on inside past the No Admittance sign. Shocked to see civilians walk into that inner sanctum, three scrubs-clad staff turned to face us through a window in the wall.

"This is Aaron Hall's mom," Nancy said. "Dr. Cusimano left her a note that Aaron is supposed to be in NICU, and he isn't. No one seems to know where he is."

My teeth chattered. The tight belt of nausea around my middle had me nearly doubled over. Chest heaving, gripping my belly, I was a deer in headlights, and the car was still coming. The note, the note, Dr. Cusimano sent the note. Where the hell did I put the note? It had my kid's name on it. I dropped my bag on the floor to fish for it. *Aaron survived, right? He couldn't have died after the surgeon left, could he?*

"Humph." Someone — could have been a nurse, a doctor, the maintenance person (they all wore standard green scrubs and immaculate Crocs) scanned a list. "He was done a long time ago." She stepped a few strides to her right and peered down an interior corridor. "Is that him?" she said, pointing, and then realizing I couldn't see where she was pointing. She came around and held open the swinging door with the circular window in it — think restaurant kitchen door — and I peeked my head into the pristine white hallway. About twenty feet down the hall there was a gurney pulled to the side, with no one around, and there he was, a blood-soaked pillow behind his head, his face turned to the side away from me, his nearly black curls spilling over the top of the mattress, as I came up beside him.

As if on cue, or because someone became aware (was alerted?) that a civilian was walking around the surgical suites, a few scrubs-wearing folks came out of a room nearby. *Surgical team? Security?*

"This is my son." It was a declaration, a claim staked, and if I'd been able, I would have drawn my weapon on the sons of bitches that left my terrified kid alone in a hallway after a multi-hour surgical procedure on his head, with most of his face wrapped in a swath of gauze.

"We were just waiting for someone to transport him upstairs," a thirtysomething bearded guy said to me.

"How long were you gonna wait?" I asked.

"I guess we could take him to ICU ourselves," one of them said to the others. *Yeah, how about that good idea.* I walked back to where Nancy stood as two of them came to the head and the foot of the gurney, and I said, only half under my breath, "Oh, that's okay, he's just a sixteen-year-old kid who had brain surgery ... No need to rush him to intensive care."

I'll never know how long Aaron waited in that hallway alone.

After they "got him settled" and allowed me in, I found him inside a glass-walled cubicle with doors that I imagined would make the *shwoop shwoop* sounds of the early Starship Enterprise. *Beam me up, Scotty.* Come to that, the entire place was so high-tech it was actually like something out of sci-fi. Aaron slept on an elevated hospital bed, bare chested, head tilted forward by a rolled blanket under his neck, his lower face obscured by a two-inch-wide strip of gauze taped under his nose, discoloured with yellow fluid and a small patch of brown blood. His skin was pale blue, his long legs were wrapped in compression stockings, and his eyes were tightly shut, like he was squeezing them hard against the pain.

"He's my son," I said breathlessly to the nurse bent over the small desk on wheels near Aaron's bed. She looked up and said nothing. Her nametag said NICU and some name that started with a *D.* I went straight to him, laying my hand on his chest. His breathing was faster than normal, and he felt surprisingly hot given his pallor.

He opened his eyes.

"Hi, buddy."

"Hi, Mom," he croaked, wincing at throat pain. "Am I okay?"

"You are."

Dr. Cusimano came up to the other side of the bed and smiled down at his patient. "You did well, Aaron. It was a long day, but you're doing great." He rested his hand on Aaron's arm just above the two intravenous lines that were secured by large square bandages. They pulled the hairs on his arms taut, and I wondered if it hurt.

"The blood pressure?" Dr. Cusimano said, looking to the nurse and back to the small blood-pressure monitor behind Aaron's head. Then I looked at the numbers for the first time.

"Oh my God," I said out loud. Aaron's blood pressure was 190 over 145. "When will that come down?" I asked to the room.

"It should be down by now," Dr. Cusimano said. Was he accusing the nurse or just being officious? He turned to the nurse again. "What are we giving him for pain?"

I was staring at dime-sized red spots I'd just noticed across Aaron's chest, shoulders, and creeping up his neck. "What's that?"

"Morphine," the nurse said, coming to the doctor's side. "He's reacting. We need to switch to fentanyl." She grabbed a small bag, rushing to hang it on the IV pole, leaving the morphine line to drop to the floor. She pulled a black Sharpie from her pocket and began circling the red hives so that they could see any changes.

"I'll do that for you," I said, and she passed me the marker. I circled all the ones I could see, as fast as I could. The beeping on one of the monitors slowed down a minute later. Aaron's heart rate was slowing. I knew from experience this meant his pain was lessening. Dr. Cusimano stood with his hands in his pockets, letting the nurse move around him, then stepped out to check on another patient. The automatic blood-pressure cuff inflated and deflated, and I saw that the numbers on the blood-pressure monitor weren't coming down. All I could do was watch my son's chest rise and fall.

The red splotches continued to spread. Aaron was reacting to the fentanyl too. The nurse conferred with the attending NICU physician, Dr. Jacks, and then hung a bag of Demerol, and with a red marker, circled the latest crop of hives. Aaron's blood pressure was still elevated, the top number over 170. I stood back while a nurse rushed in and out of the room, each time with something else in her hands and a marker in her mouth.

"It must be his age." Dr. Jacks said. "Young bodies react quickly to opioids."

Dr. Cusimano came in again. "Aaron, how do you feel?"

My hand was pressed over my mouth, waiting for him to speak.

Aaron opened his eyes again. Fighting what I hoped was only grogginess and not unconsciousness. "Okay. Thirsty," he replied in his scratchy voice.

"We'll get you a drink as soon as things settle down. Can you tell me what hurts?" Dr. Cusimano touched location after location on Aaron's head. Each time Aaron said, "No."

Eventually, and I don't know how much later, the blood-pressure numbers came down and Aaron's heart rate stabilized. The hives faded, leaving the black and red marker circles on his pale torso. I watched from behind a curtain of tears as Michael Cusimano, renowned brain surgeon and father of a teenage son himself, leaned in and whispered, "If you were my boy, I'd want to tell you how very proud of you I am right now."

I mouthed *thank you* to him as he left.

Justin and Rick came not long after. After coming bedside for a moment, Rick stood outside the cubicle so Justin could see Aaron; the nurse had tersely informed them "only one of you at a time." I pointed Justin to a chair a few feet inside the sliding doors and he sat down, his hands tucked under his legs. Aaron was sleeping and I stood at his shoulder. I looked at Justin and smiled, but hadn't said anything yet, not wanting to inspire the nurse to remove him.

"Mom," Justin whispered. I looked over at him, surprised by his stricken expression. "Is Aaron dead?"

My breath caught in my throat. *How could I have missed this?* Justin couldn't see Aaron's chest, didn't know the beeping was actually monitoring Aaron's breathing, and judging only by the strained look on my face, Justin thought he'd lost his brother. In the melee, where Rick and I had been shuttling the kid around like a suitcase all day, we hadn't bothered to tell him his brother had come through. So far, anyway.

"No, buddy, he's alive," I told him. "He's alive."

Justin's face crumpled in relief.

When I called my parents with the news, I was unsurprised to hear my mother scold that it was about time I called. "You know that I've been beside myself with worry all day!" she fumed. I had déjà vu; those were practically the same words out of her mouth when Aaron had hernia surgery at a couple of months old. The cauldron within me, which had simmered my entire life, boiled over again, and it humiliated me that at forty-three years old, I had no stinging words to hurl back at her. I wanted to yell, "Do you have any idea what we've been through?" or "Even now, you can only think of yourself?" On this worst of days, it flayed me open that my mother didn't ask what was happening with Justin or whether we needed help. She didn't offer the customary, "Is there something I can do?" After a couple of *Thank Gods*, she rushed to get off the phone to call some friend at the church with the good news. I resigned myself to let Kelly do the updating from there on in.

Aaron's vital signs did not co-operate or stabilize for long that afternoon or into the evening. We were allowed brief visits and then we were shooed out by the nurse. I asked politely if one of us could stay — "He's only sixteen" — and I got the well-rehearsed speech about rules and was told they would call us if there was any change. Any change? There had been constant change. Aaron was dozing, but he was thirsty constantly and had questions, and he was just a freaking kid. In the evening, I pulled Dr. Cusimano aside to ask if there was anything he could do to get us permission to stay with Aaron through this first night. He said he would most certainly speak to the nurse, and within moments of his moving on to another patient, she approached me standing at the bedrail and said flatly, "People don't have visitors here." I understood that this was a top-level facility, which served trauma patients from across a vast region, and I wasn't accustomed to being pressed out of the way, but an internal voice I prefer not to heed told me to pick my battles and not to make enemies among this NICU nursing staff, so I backed down. This was a hospital for adults, and no accommodations were going to be made for a teenager who wanted his mother. My fury was nearly irrepressible. Rick patiently listened to my rant, and as always, together, we made a new plan.

We couldn't stay in the room with our boy, so Rick slept in a chair outside the intensive care unit, visiting Aaron when he woke (when he was allowed), and I drove Justin home, nearly nodding off in my own exhaustion, trying to scare myself into the wakefulness that I needed to get my youngest son home safely, while I left my prone, terrified older son in the hands of strangers. I hated it all.

Aaron still tells stories of how upset he was that night, of having intense headaches, being thirsty and hungry and not wanting to ask for anything except Mom. And being told I'd left.

Home with Justin fed and asleep, I tended to our animals, told my sister what was happening in a quick phone call, texted with Rick to get an update, and fell into my bed, fully clothed, to grab a few hours sleep.

But I had a new mantra: *He's still here.*

14

PERSONAL SUPPORT WORKER

The following day Aaron was moved to a private room on the critical-care floor, just steps outside of the NICU where Rick and I had felt not just unwelcome but almost forbidden, unable to be by Aaron's side. And Aaron kept reminding us of this. He complained tearfully about the night before, holding me responsible for not being there, even accusing me of lying to him. I'd wished that he would sleep most of the time and not know he was alone, but it didn't play out that way. The noises, interruptions, bright lights, and attentive staff had him on alert through the night, aware of the terror, remembering television shows and movie scenes. And abandonment inflamed his anxiety.

During the nighttime routine of passing by their beds when they were little, I would sometimes stand over them, see their eyelids flickering in REM, little blue veins flashing like fireflies in summer. They were safe, secure, hope-filled. Or is it that I was hope-filled and they were just not burned by the world yet?

Now I stood over a different bed, absorbing the details of a man-sized face I had feared I might never watch sleeping again. I counted the minutes of rest and mentally noted the quality of his sleep. Someone would ask me later. I checked the fluid levels on his catheter bag, monitored exactly how much he'd had to drink, and answered every question the medical staff had about him. When he dozed, I memorized him, again. Hope was in that room and I was having trouble claiming it, but I could patrol the perimeter until he was well enough to walk out of there.

I was out getting Aaron food, a couple of blocks away at the Toronto Eaton Centre, when Rick called my cell saying Dr. Cusimano wanted to talk to us.

About another surgery. They needed to go in again.

"Does Aaron know?" I asked, tears starting. My legs were moving under me, negotiating around columns of people pouring out of the Queen Street subway station.

"Not yet. Dr. Cusimano said we'll all talk about it together when you get here. Hurry."

It was smart to go back in while Aaron was still in hospital, hadn't begun healing yet, and the entire surgical team was present for a repeat of the day before. But how was I going to tell Aaron? Where the heck would I find the words? "I know you just went through the most horrific experience of your life, but now you have to do it again. Today."

He brightened a little when I rushed into the hospital room, a Burger King bag under my arm. It seemed only seconds later Dr. Cusimano joined us around Aaron's bed. Aaron looked as much a little boy as ever. But the size of his head and face and feet hanging over the end of the bed would have made this comical to anyone else (they had removed the footboard since they couldn't find a bed extender — the hospital had only two). "How many patients do you have who are six and a half feet tall?" I'd asked the head nurse, jokingly. "You'd be surprised," she said. "There's a basketball team in this city, after all."

I remained conflicted. Going to an experienced surgeon, going to Cusimano meant foregoing whatever emotional and psychological comfort Aaron might have gained by being at a pediatric hospital. It wasn't just about him fitting into the bed, it was also about him fitting in, being treated like the scared kid he was, by people in a place where the culture boasted it was committed to kids and their families. Should I have found some way to have him operated on at SickKids? Should I have asked the doctors to work together, insisted that he be in a child-centred environment? Maybe I hadn't tried hard enough. The beds were going to be too short, regardless, but they never treated him with the extra compassion and attentiveness that I felt a kid in a hospital deserved. But I could not doubt the surgeon who stood with his hand resting on my son's shoulder and began, "We think there is benefit in going in again, Aaron. We'd like to operate again tomorrow." Aaron's eyes locked on mine, cutting through me, accusing me, blaming me, begging me. I would not let myself look away. Cusimano tracked Aaron's gaze to me, and reading the tension, he offered, "I talked to your parents about this yesterday."

I wish he hadn't said that.

I'd known this was a possibility. And now Aaron realized I'd kept this from him. That this was what he'd told me to do didn't matter. I had to be the parent now. We'd be sidekicks later, and I might never have a chance to fix the cleft in our relationship if the surgery did not go well. Lose. Lose. Lose.

One of our family rules — a promise is a promise — came instinctively to my defence, but I couldn't use it, couldn't let him know that I understood the ridicule and rage and betrayal he was feeling. I needed him to muster the courage to do this. I had to stand by my plan to only tell him what he asked to know, but this seemed like no-rules-apply territory. Rick and I had crouched over two computer screens the day before in the nurses' station, where four surgeons toggled back and forth from pre-surgical CT scans and MRIs to post-surgical views. Rick and I had leaned in, squinting for some grey patch the doctors assured us was tumour, surrounded by innumerable other grey-ish shapes that fit inside what was obviously my boy's cranium. There is no objectivity when it is your child's scan. Even if our untrained eyes could locate whatever the hell Dr. Cusimano was asking us to see, we did not want to find it, not really. There was never going to be a day when I would glance at a screen and exclaim, "Oh look, isn't that fascinating! A great big tumour in my son's head." I didn't want to identify the residual tumour, I wanted to scoop up our child, swaddle him the way I did when he was a newborn, and run out of the NICU as if I'd pulled off a bank heist. *Please, not my baby … Please, not my baby …* pounding its relentless rhythm through my head as I looked away from the monitors, willing the tears to wait just a few more minutes to preserve some amount of dignity. I could not fathom this was happening. We were calmly talking to a team of brain surgeons about operating on my sixteen-year-old son again. *How is this not a sci-fi movie?*

Rick and I, parents but no longer partners, a successful cor-porate executive and an urban designer turned author, stood like useless space-holders, pylons. What could we say about the speculation that another microscopic adventure behind my son's face could improve the chances of grasping another minute piece of tumour? "Every cell we take improves the chances that the secreting portions of the adenoma have been excised."

"Uh-huh," was what I managed back.

"We feel there is a good chance that we can get a bit more of the remnant. We only got about sixty percent of it in the pro-cedure. Please think about it, and we'll let you know how things look after another follow-up MRI."

Now looking down at Aaron's swollen face, the massive strips of tape stretching under his nose holding globs of blood-soaked packing in his nostrils, his eyes told me how scared he was at the thought of going into surgery again.

Dr. Cusimano, in a tender gesture, moved closer, bent at the waist and took Aaron's hand in his two. "I know this isn't what you might have wanted. I'll leave you to talk to your parents about it, but we need to know in the next few minutes."

Dr. Cusimano had barely pulled the door closed when Aaron, blotchy skinned, wet-eyed, and pursed mouthed looked up into my face, and spit his terror at me. "I'll hate you forever if you make me do this."

And I ran.

I felt like I'd been jabbed with a red-hot poker in the belly. Turning right out of his room, I covered the short distance to the elevator and elbowed my way through the people getting on, then two at a time ran down the steps into the Toronto street. I just kept running, the thrumming of "Oh my God, oh my God" coming out of my mouth in rhythm with my feet on the sidewalk. I heard as much as felt long breaths drawing up through my nose, and then the tightening of my chest. *Jesus, I'm going to have a heart attack.*

My phone vibrated in my pocket. I ignored it. *He hates me for this.* I walked. *I did this to him.* I kept walking. *Where am I going now?* I couldn't go back. *How am I going to face him again? My son hates me.* Pulled, more than pushed, I walked up the middle of the wide concrete steps, treading on hollows worn down from a century of use, and into the vestibule of the massive church beside the hospital. Conscious of my heaving chest and a sound coming out of me like a wounded animal, I put my hand over my mouth as I tucked into a pew halfway down the sanctuary. *What an appropriate name,* I thought. *Sanctuary: safe haven, calm in the storm, place of hiding.*

A half-dozen other people dotted the space. One lit a candle at the front, another two bowed their heads together whispering prayers, and others knelt on the padded rails. I stared up at the architecture, the history, and begged the stained glass windows to give me the strength to walk this path alone. He'd come through the first one. *Have faith for God's sake!* He'll come through and be better for it the second time. An impossible but obvious choice. I hadn't come into that church for God. I was seeking a place where I could work out in my mind how doing the right thing for my kid could come with such a price ... his life, his love, my heart.

A different woman walked out of that church. I'd never be able to reassemble myself now. I carried self-loathing and self-criticism with me out those doors, added to the healthy dose of blame I already accepted for ruining my family. I was always going to be afraid. Of everything. This was my punishment, to lose my confidence, to always know I could be shattered by a threat to my children, by a terse word from them. I laid my backbone on the altar in that church and didn't care if I ever found it again.

I glanced at my phone, at a text from Rick. He wants to say he's sorry. He needs you to come back.

I still can't. I'm a mess.

Take your time. He's good now.

Damn it all, what if they need me there to say yes. I can't stay away.

There was the rub again, and Aaron's operating room time could be forfeited if even a single member of his surgical team left early for the weekend. I had to go back right away. If the signing authority thing came up, if they needed Aaron to sign and he refused, the legal responsibility fell to me. Irony is a bitch. He may never forgive me but I was still going to have to do the rational parent thing and make the call, one that could cost me my son.

I might lose him either way.

Very early the next morning, while I was still dabbing my sore eyes and licking my proverbial wounds, Aaron was wheeled away from us into the operating room. Again. This time, he went without anxiety and without fear.

Instead, he'd tried some comedy. "Look at Mom, you'd think she was the one having surgery."

Rick looked at me pityingly. I mustered a smile. The tears dripped down my cheeks. I could not remember forcing my son to do even the smallest thing, including room cleanup or airing his hockey equipment. I'd never forced Santa pictures, lining up to shake the hands of famous sports players, or command performances on piano … and there I was giving him no way out of having a life-risking surgery. Again. I seethed at myself. I avoided eye contact with him. It was all I could do just to keep breathing.

"I'm not even feeling nervous now," he boasted. Rick and I smiled. We'd been through sleepless days, seeing him in pain, watching him fast, seeing him try to stand up only to lose his balance, and listening to his anguish over not being able to breathe through his nose because of the packing. We were running an endurance race on an unpredictable course that meandered around him while he walked the shorter, straighter line of healing. We got two days under our belts, and it was all going to start over now. The nurses, anesthesiologists, and assisting surgeons came by his bed in pre-op and took his blood pressure, ticked their checklists, and cross-referenced hospital bracelets and birth dates. No elevated blood pressure, fidgetiness, or blotchy red face. Aaron was calm facing surgery. I paced like a caged lion, fighting nausea, the self-talk on repeat in my head. Rick stood, arms crossed, leaning against the wall beside Aaron's pillows. Our boy looked so comfortable in the situation at that moment that it would not have surprised me if he flung his long legs over the side of the bed and went over to chat up other patients.

I know that we didn't wait as long on that day, but I remember nothing else. The immediate recovery from his second surgery, the aftermath, is gone for me, partitioned off in the place in my mind where events I can't face remain. The second surgery was considered a failure. I'm certain they never said those words to me, but I'm also certain I read them in a report somewhere, at some point later. They didn't get the rest of the tumour. They didn't get any more at all. Aaron would have to deal with the disease for the rest of his life. This meant another round of intense Google diving. Living with gigantism into adulthood left questions that I'd hoped to avoid — Would he get to do all the things he wanted to? What would his life be like? How long would he live?

Gigantism and its clinical cousin, acromegaly, are not sexy media-darling topics in the illness world. This means they are not discussed as often or understood as well by laypeople as things like heart disease or the better-known cancers. There are not vast tomes published for clinicians and patients offering treatment and management strategies.

In Aaron's case, tests concluded that most of the hormones produced by his pituitary gland were either deficient or decreased, called panhypopituitarism. Most significantly, Aaron's growth hormone was more than thirty-five times what it should have been in a prepubescent person. But other pituitary hormones were very low, predicting the serious delay in puberty's onset. The definitive evaluation tool for gigantism and acromegaly is the measurement of a hormone called insulin-like growth factor 1 (IGF-1). Aaron's had been 1,357 when first tested, and the goal (although his doctors opinions varied) was for it to be in the 200s, and relatively quickly, if treatment was to be considered successful. Post-op blood tests were repeated frequently and it had been remarkable to watch his growth hormone and

IGF-1 levels drop just hours after the first surgery, and whether it was due to weight loss from lack of solid food (almost twenty pounds in ten days) or the surgical results, his facial appearance was drastically altered.

Of course, he wanted to hear none of this. If it's possible for hearing to be turned off, Aaron managed it in those days when I was asking for the latest numbers. I wanted him out of the hospital, and I was hoping he wouldn't need supplemental medication, but his creature comforts were foremost for him, as were the events going on around him. "I couldn't believe it, Mom. Some woman came in and asked where my wife was." I chose to see the compliment in this ... that I looked young enough to be the partner of anyone younger than my forty-three years, but I didn't try to be funny each time he told me that something else had happened when I dared to leave his room. His anger and anxiety were understandable, but I was starting to wonder if I was rationalizing something I should have been making more of. He was moody. Really moody.

Mike and Nancy had mentioned this about Brendan. They weren't willing to dismiss it as teenage self-aggrandizement in the months after surgery, and this stayed with me. What if Aaron's affect was going to be different, his personality somewhat altered? We hadn't been warned about that, but with so few patients with the disease, so little experience of this for any one surgeon, was anyone even considering how surgery on a pituitary tumour might impact a patient's psychology? But I couldn't think about that right then. Just like when I brought him home as an infant, we had to deal with basic needs first.

He was so hungry. "Why can't I have real food? Can't I please have something that requires chewing? I'm tired of drinking my food! When can I use a straw?"

And he still had his IV and a catheter, which he hated. Precautions were in place in case he needed to be rushed back into surgery because of an infection, bleed, inflammation, or spinal leak, among the other things they rhymed off while he slept. "He's sixteen. Can we please talk in the hallway?"

I was mostly glad of how expressive he was. I said *mostly.* "Aaron is a talker," Rick and I always said to one another. I cringed to think how long the tumour might have had to wreak havoc if Aaron hadn't told me about his head, his knees, and agonizingly, his fears. But when you welcome the rain, sometimes you get a torrent. He couldn't get comfortable in the bed. He needed to have his head elevated. He could feel "disgusting shit" running down the back of his throat. The lights were too bright. "Why is everything so dark? Is it nighttime?" He was too big. The "stupid" bed was too small. After his second surgery, he was in a standard-issue bed with a fixed footboard, so he was forced to sleep with his knees up (while on his back, since he was not supposed to lie on his side).

He'd been lying on his back around the clock for days when an athletically-built woman with tight black curls came into his room one afternoon, saying, "Hi, I'm Mindy and I'm getting you out of that bed."

"I don't want to," Aaron grumbled, looking at me, not her.

"Well, you can't go home until you can walk," Mindy said. And she marched up to the side of the bed, pushing a wheelchair with one hand and pulling a walker with the other. I offered to help. "Leave it to me," she said genially, positioning herself. She bent her powerful legs and hauled my 240-pound son up from his hospital bed. It had been four days, and he had only tentatively tried to stand up once before. He was really scared he'd fall and hit his head or hurt someone.

"Lean on me, I've got you," she said.

"Yeah right, you're smaller than my mother."

"Son," she said, her left hand splayed open on his sternum, making him look into her face, "I will not let anything happen to you. Put your arms around my shoulders and shuffle your feet. I've got your bag." She slung his urine-output bag over her arm on a hook, and he did exactly what she said. Tears dribbled off the end of my nose. He was up.

She was a force of freaking nature, this woman. Unrelenting. Always with a quip, a comment, ready for any mood he brought, as if she had met dozens of bleary teenagers suffering from the post-op blues. Mindy got Aaron to a chair (she quickly realized the wheelchair would not accommodate him, and I dragged in the sleeper chair I'd been using).

"I'll be back in a few hours and help you back to bed."

"You're just gonna leave me here?" he asked her back as she hurried out. Peeking her head back into the room, she whispered, "You can use those legs anytime you want, ya know. They operated on your head, and it's a looong way away from your legs."

I couldn't stop grinning.

In those days, it was so common for hospital staff to come into Aaron's room and walk past his elderly roommate (ignoring the shouts of the constantly complaining old fella) that I didn't offer much by way of greeting. I had long since exhausted my patience with the impersonal. I glanced up from my journal when a man in his thirties with striking blue eyes, impeccably dressed, like a dutiful prep-school attendee, came to Aaron's bedside. He had the two-inch blue binder, Aaron's chart, in his hand. I said nothing. They mostly came and looked, smiled at me, and read Aaron's chart while my son pretended to sleep or gave them the stink eye. Dr. Watkins introduced himself then added, "I was part of Aaron's surgical team."

Aaron's eyes flew open.

Dr. Watkins moved closer to Aaron's shoulder. "Can we talk about how you feel?" My lump of teenager did not reply. "Can you tell me how this all started, Aaron?" Aaron's long finger pointed at me. It was story time. I started the spiel.

"A CT scan showed a 3.6 centimetre tumour three months ago."

"It really was enormous!" Dr. Watkins said, remembering from the operating room, I assumed, but he sounded like a kid just off the Ferris wheel.

He asked about medications as he flipped from one divided section of the heavy blue binder to another. "We don't have that information here."

I pointed to the little laptop beside me. "Do you need me to give it to you?" I couldn't believe Aaron was an in-patient in a major hospital and the doctors were coming to the kid's mom for a medication list.

"While you're finding that, do you know what the date of his last MRI was?"

I looked up. I wanted to say, *You're kidding me right? Do you not have a hundred pages of information right there in your hands?* I imagined myself a different kind of mother, more like my own mother would be in this situation. I tried envisioning myself getting puffed up and big, leaning across the bed, poking a firm finger into the middle of the doctor's chest and shouting — no, *growling* — "Look it up!" But I only replied with medication names, dosages, and dates, and added, "I have an electronic copy if you'd like that too."

"We are very pleased with how things went." *Uh-huh. Eight of you stood over my son, clipping tumour remnants and pulling them out through tubes inserted through his nostrils. That must have been a real treat.*

"How do you feel, Aaron?"

"Okay."

"That's it?" They both looked at me.

And I stepped in, partly so my kid wouldn't be presumed to be rude (mom instinct) and partly because a freaking brain surgeon was in the room and we needed this assessment. "Aaron, he wants you to tell him about your head, gut, pee, mouth, nose, whatever seems like a problem to you."

He stared up at me, eyes wet with tears, and then dropped his head back onto the pillow to look up at the ceiling.

"My nose is so sore. The blood dripping onto my lip is disgusting. I don't think I'll ever eat again. I hate being stuck in this bed. I can't feel my butt anymore. Why are there little black wires coming out of my head and how freaking long will this catheter be in? The old man in the bed next to me moans and groans all night and doesn't smell that great, and" — lifting his head to look at Dr. Watkins — "were you there when they got the tumour? I don't remember seeing you when they put me to sleep."

With a shared grin and a giggle, I reminded Dr. Watkins, "You wanted details."

And it hit me: *This is what my life is now.* Urge him, translate for him, remember the details, see things he doesn't. *What does this make me?* More Than Mom.

Don't mistake this for a sweet story about the intimate bond of mutual trust that would be possible for another mom and son. Moms of toddlers who scream, "Nooo!" when they lean in for a kiss would smile at this illustration of the older boy who trusts and needs his mom to be his voice. Those moms would hope that a bond would prevail through challenging times. Moms of almost-adult men will remember when their teenage sons wouldn't speak for themselves whether stubborn or lazy, when they hear about Aaron and me, and bless them. They will remember the last vestiges of being this essential to their sons' daily lives. Illness put a filter on this scene. The way that Aaron and I tag teamed wasn't ever going to be a classic Mom-can't-let-go. We accepted that a line had been crossed, and like we were in a three-legged race, we were going to have to find a tolerance and a rhythm to move forward.

Dr. Watkins took time to answer each question and spoke to Aaron, guy to guy. I hoped he wouldn't go into more details than Aaron wanted, and when he started in about how Aaron's nose was sore because the instruments put pressure on the nostrils and what the liquid from his nose actually was, I cringed. But the visual of what the heavy-gauge threads coming from the back of his head were for — stitches with the tails left long — was more than even I could take. I turned away as he explained very briefly that a patient's head has to be held very still during surgery, and I silently prayed to myself that Aaron would lose interest with the surgical technique at that moment.

"I'll need your help with this," Dr. Watkins said to me.

"Of course." He handed me a small blue basin, the kind that people throw up in. "I think we're going to get the packing out of there for you, Aaron."

While I managed my heaving guts, this meticulously dressed man used oversized plastic tweezers and pulled blood and mucous and packing soaked with God knows what from Aaron's nostrils. Without the huge strip of gauze taped under his nose, I saw that his nostrils were swollen to the diameter of a nickel each. As Dr. Watkins pulled, the packing snaked into the basin; once in a while he would stop to pack it down so that another length could be pulled and laid there without spilling over onto Aaron's bedding.

I was almost gagging, and Aaron *was* gagging, tears rolling down his face, his eyes pinched shut.

"Is this hurting, Aaron?" My voice quavered. I was as tense as a rolling pin, and felt like I'd rip the tweezers out of the man's hand if this was hurting my kid.

"No, it's just gross. Please hurry."

Estimates on the length of packing vary, and I've learned that packing isn't always used post-operatively anymore, but Aaron liked asking the doctors who poked their heads into this room over the next day how many feet were in there. Guesses of twenty-four feet were common. But he could breathe through his nose now, and that made the next milestone inevitable.

Aaron really wanted a shower. He'd been in a bed for five days, and when I suggested they offer me a large basin and a hand cloth (I'd been trained in how to give a bed bath by my mother), a nurse said, "You could do that or you could just take him down the hall to the shower." They weren't going to do it. As if to drive the stake into my disappointment and discomfort further, she added, "You are the mother, right?"

I could push him in a wheelchair to the door. He'd be uncomfortable, but it wasn't far, and then he'd have to transfer to a bath chair. *But if he falls, all 240 pounds of him.* And I hadn't seen my son naked since he was a little boy. He was neither a man whose wife could assist him nor a little child.

"Dude, we're going to have to figure out how to do this together."

And like so many things before, we got it done. I was intent on not violating his privacy and scarring our dented relationship any further. And I didn't want to lead him to believe he would always need my help or give him the impression that he wasn't healing well or quickly enough. I had to find a way. Using handrails on the wall, he got himself seated in the shower on a supportive chair. He peeled away his hospital gown, and while I turned away, he covered himself with a towel. I stood shoeless in the small space and pointed the shower down onto him while he put his hands on my waist to support himself when he felt like he was leaning. Just as the water was pouring over his hair and he put his head back a little so the translucent stream could veil his face, I glanced down to ensure I wouldn't step on his toes. I gasped. Our feet were in an inch of bloody water.

"Oh God, A-man, you're bleeding." He reached a hand up to where long wiry sutures hung from the back of his head, now obvious because his hair was flattened and wet.

I looked to where the emergency-call cord hung on the wall. Could I reach it without letting Aaron fall onto the tile floor?

I pulled his head to me and gently picked the hair away from the scabs where the surgical pins had been. The incision points were pink. Maybe it wasn't fresh blood. I looked down again; the water at our feet was lightening in colour. And as we froze there in our pose, connected yet separate, the mom and son we were and the two people we would be now, we let the water carry away everything that had happened this week, and we both sobbed. I washed and rewashed his hair like when he was a little boy, and perhaps because he felt the shower hid his tears or because it was only me there, he let it all out.

15

PUNCHING BAG

Around the time that our surgery date got moved ahead, we had heard that Aaron's friend Randy, who'd been battling cancer, was in palliative care. And now he'd lost his fight, and his mother was burying her son. I had no right to feel any kinship with Randy's mother, yet wisps of anguish encircled me like smoke from an abandoned cigarette as we lined up at the wake. I looked up at Rick. I was ashamed to be thinking of my own kid. Were all the other parents thinking of theirs too?

The boys hadn't seen each other, nor had we parents spoken, in months, each confronting our own unthinkable. Our kids had been in class together and on the same teams for years. I was on the bench at the hockey game acting as trainer when Randy had begun throwing up and needed me to take him to the dressing room. His parents said he was dealing with anxiety, explaining that he got worked up on the ice. Two years later we stood at his funeral.

I don't know if Randy's family knew that this was Aaron's first, wobbly, head-pounding outing. How could they? The same days when I could very well have lost my son in surgery in one hospital, Randy's mother was watching her boy fade across the city.

Aaron insisted we remove the gauze and tape from beneath his nose and I jammed a Kleenex in his pocket just in case. He wouldn't be able to stand long enough for the funeral, so we made sure he could attend the wake. As Aaron greeted his other friends there, we heard their surprised comments that Aaron was "out" and "looked okay." They'd heard he had cancer too. Because he'd left school without telling anyone, they thought he was terminal. That was gut-punch irony. I'd confront this in the rare-disease world continually in the years to come. People think only cancer kills. They don't know that medical monsters take children's lives wearing many clinical costumes. There are over seven thousand rare diseases, and while some of them are cancers, the majority are less well-known life-takers and quality-of-life killers too.

This could have been us. This could have been us. The realization throbbed in my head and I was embarrassed to be crying so hard. In days since he'd come through surgery, I'd waded back into the shallow safety of denial. I'd wrapped myself in some it's-okay-now cushioning, but the wake was like a cold shower.

At the funeral days later, Rick and I cried to the sound of country music playing. Miley Cyrus's "The Climb" became the lament of every sick child — Randy, Aaron, and every child who deserves to live a longer life. Grief and strain poured out of us. We cried for what we'd been through. We cried for Randy's family. For their loss. For ourselves. For my deep wish for a do-over, the marriage, the boys' childhoods, Aaron's last few months. There, leaning into one another in the standing-room-only church, we bled out in a broad shaft of white sunlight teeming through the stained glass windows.

Outside we spoke to kind hockey coaches and teachers who asked in whispers about Aaron, who they had heard was pulled out of school for health reasons. Rick and I tried to brush off questions with responses inviting folks to call us or Aaron himself because that day was not about Aaron. When Randy's father, Dave, hugged me, speaking thanks softly in my ear, I saw pure grace in his demeanour. I would never be able to manage so well.

About three weeks after surgery, Aaron was bright, chatty, and funny again, reflecting back on the surgeries, hospitals, doctors, and caregivers at an appointment in Dr. Kirsch's office. His moodiness had faded away. He even brought up (with more than a little pride) how he had teased me before his second surgery, that I had been more afraid than he. I was too tender to banter on that subject, and he took full advantage. He told Dr. Kirsch that his relationship with me didn't fare too well on the day that the decision about the second surgery was made, and then turning his eyes on me asked, "But we're okay now, aren't we, Mom?"

Yes, son, we're okay.

Homeschooling began about the same time. The vice-principal and I had met to make arrangements to hire teachers to support Aaron's completion of Grade 10 Math, Science, and French. She'd been enthusiastic about homeschooling, reminding me that because Aaron was a good student there was a great deal of leniency at her discretion. Aaron got a pass for his physical-education credit, but the core courses had to be completed to a satisfactory level or he would lose the semester's progress and be held back. The future looked uncertain and dour already, and I didn't want him to face being delayed completing high school. When the tutors began working with him, we all realized (and perhaps were forced to remember) that his brain had been impacted by the surgery. He was exhausted and not able to focus his attention in the first few sessions, but he improved steadily over a few weeks.

In addition to our follow-up medical appointments, we did some day trips, drive-ins, and summer-release films. I finally took time to nest a little in the new house, adding a few pieces of outdoor furniture and having the boys' rooms painted the primary colours they'd insisted on. Pressed on by the desire that there would be some highlights for him, some good times while Justin carried on with sports camps, Aaron and I did other things like the zoo, the mall, and *a lot* of restaurants. That summer baseball games became a natural for us. It was tough to cram Aaron's long legs into a regular seat at the stadium, but we found that if I kept my legs tightly crossed and over to one side, my extra legroom became his, and he could manage. And the food came to the seats! Between innings at one game, we were standing just behind the accessible seating area, cramming our mouths with huge overpriced hotdogs, when I felt stares, not at me but at Aaron. Out of the corner of my eye I saw a man just a few feet away turn in his seat to face us. He was about sixty and was sitting beside an older woman and a twentysomething woman, who was next to a young man in a wheelchair. The young woman raised her hand to her mouth while staring at my boy and said, "Oh my God, oh my God," in a tone that was somewhere between horror and disgust. All four of them were looking back and forth at one another, exchanging whispered words and glances. I felt the heat rise in my face. Not the sting of tears, the heat of anger.

I looked at Aaron. He was completely aware of it.

"Just let it go, Mom." He was looking away, as if they didn't exist, eating his hot dog and staring out over the blue metal railing. "It happens all the time. I'm used to it."

"You shouldn't have to be." It was so close and so blatant, the rudest gawking I'd been through with him. This felt like we were in a ring at the circus.

Something defiant rose in me, emerged out of me. "What are you lookin' at?" I said loudly. Then, before turning, I looked directly at the man in the wheelchair. "You know what, I would've expected better from someone who must get treated like this all the time." I touched the back of Aaron's arm and steered us into the crowd.

Stigma was in our lives now. Aaron was managing way better than I was. He didn't entertain the questions, however polite. He rebuffed them unless a child asked. Kids were amazed by his height because they saw something else, because they didn't contrast Aaron to their self-image. He was not different than them, he was marvelous.

I wished I could protect him from the gauntlet of public opinion, of stigma and social obstacles, which could leave the most indelible wounds.

There was something I could do though ... I called it Aaron-proofing. I remembered how new parents were told to childproof for their commando crawling babes. Get down on the floor and have a look at what baby might put in their mouth, pick up and eat, or bonk their head on. The places I looked were just higher. I looked up for the same purpose young parents look down. I'd gauge the number of inches that the hydraulic housing on an automatic door hung down. Aaron would duck a little, but if he didn't scan ahead, he'd get Smartied. (Hitting your head on the little round button on the top of a baseball cap, in Canadian parlance, is "getting Smartied.") There was never a time that he didn't have a ball cap on at that age, so this was a real concern. He'd get hit when I closed the sunroof, or by a low hanging light fixture, and by decorations at Christmas.

The world of average-sized people reminded him of his difference — his exceptionality (my preferred) — from the moment he got up in the morning. Correction: Even his bed was too small for him to stretch out on. Seats on planes, suspended ceiling tiles, the tread-length on stairs, shower stalls, too-low countertops, and bottom shelves in fridges were all wrong for him.

Aaron didn't like me pointing out the obstacles. "I see it Mom!" Although sometimes we added "spot the obstacle" to our snickering repartee. "That would've taken your eye out," I said, as he moved an orange sign that dangled from hooks on the ceiling. "Well, that's ironic," he said, prompting me to look up at the sign swinging back into place: Caution. Protective Equipment Is Required in This Area. And we burst out laughing as we stepped onto the elevator.

Aaron had his own strategy, and I was catching on too — he just didn't go anywhere or see people anymore in the weeks after his time in hospital. I caught some remarks about feeling self-conscious about his low energy, his insatiable appetite and thirst (I think he was putting away five or six thousand calories a day). Litres of unwatered-down juice, stacks of sandwiches, whole pizzas (Buffalo-wing-flavoured preferred), boxes of frozen fruit bars, family-sized powdered mini-donuts, full wheels of grocery-store-prepared cut vegetables. My mother took to baking him a cake every week and barbecuing a box of hamburger patties so that Aaron could make himself a burger in the microwave between meals. There wasn't a between meals. He would feel light-headed and dizzy if he didn't eat. It wasn't sugar he needed. There was no particular craving. His body was telling him to eat, in a primal way, it seemed. His weight had restored to around two hundred pounds (he was now six foot six, managing to gain an inch, give or take, since it all began). He often asked me if I thought his weight was okay. I couldn't imagine being asked about my weight multiple times a week, like he was by techs, nurses, specialists, and the blood-work people. I finally showed him a body-mass-index calculator where he landed squarely on *normal*, and that seemed to satisfy him.

Aaron was not thin, gangly, or "spindly," as he called it. The soft-tissue bulking, the inflammation, and the weight was one of the ways to intuit (if you're medically inclined) someone who was genetically tall from someone who had acromegaly or another endocrine-related disease such as Marfan syndrome. (I wish more people knew this so they would ask Aaron fewer times if he was a basketball player.) Aaron was at the low end of the height range for players in the NBA, and although his weight quite likely comprised a much different muscle-fat ratio than theirs, he was on par.

Self-consciousness is the prerogative of teenagerhood, and I was thankful that *everyone* his age was overly self-critical, hoping this would ease his return back into social life when school began. The summer hadn't done his introversion or avoidance any favours. But Aaron's self-consciousness was neither temporary nor typical. My wishing I could place this on the short-term angst-causing list, along with acne or being thick around the middle this summer and needing a belt in the fall, was naive.

Further, he was feeling self-conscious that he wasn't healing as well as people expected him too. It took me a while of listening carefully to him to figure out that he meant his emotions, and whatever else he was ruminating on. His energy, physical capability, and body image too, perhaps, were making him feel judged, exposed, less than. It would come clear eventually, I trusted.

"I don't want Dad coming to the appointments," he said from the kitchen table when I was writing down a follow-up appointment time with one of his surgeons.

"Why?" I asked, not turning to see his face.

"He makes me feel like I'm not doing this well enough … getting better, I mean." His face was cast downward, shoulders rolled in. I didn't open my mouth to rebut or defend. "He doesn't need to come, right?" His eyebrows raised. "We've got this, right?"

I was wedged. If I agreed, I could be limiting Rick's involvement, and that could hurt him or cause him to feel I was pressing him out, and I didn't want either. If I said no, I wasn't honouring Aaron's right to choose how this all went down. "Should I just tell Dad we've got it handled?" His shoulders lowered. I wasn't going to make him go into it. Another cellmate deal made. I'd hold back details when I spoke to Rick.

"But I absolutely *don't* want my brother to come." That much, at least, hadn't changed.

Mothers have a not-so-secret superpower — we are unflappable around body fluids. I was no stranger to messes, injuries, or gross boy stuff, and we lived in the forest where they took jumps off their mountain bikes and rode courses on suspended two by fours. But I never counted on knowing what the inside of my kid's head looked like. I shouldn't have ever wondered where all that packing went, because my curiosity was satiated. His otolaryngologist ... better known to us as the ear, nose, and throat surgeon, rechecked Aaron regularly to ensure that scar tissue in his nostrils healed sufficiently to restore his full respiration. He snored now, something that would abate, she ensured us. Aaron sat back as cameras were inserted in his nostrils and breathing flow tests were done. He really enjoyed Dr. Janice, and as I've shared, that was a rarity and a welcome respite. Dr. Janice was cool and stylish and unfazed by questions, and I often wondered if her hair curled just to keep up with her. I asked her about the long sutures that were still in Aaron's hair, and in a flash she was there clipping the four-inch wiry tails off. "You won't be needing those anymore!" she said as she flung them in the garbage.

"Thank you," he said like she'd given him water after crossing the desert.

On every office visit, she'd insert a camera into his nostrils with one hand and flip the switch on a monitor with the other. I had nowhere else to look, so I watched as she guided the scope into Aaron's head, and stupidly, asked what all that was. "Oh, there's some dried sheets of mucous and scar tissue and right there is the new nose job I gave Aaron."

Mucous sheets. Ugh. I tried not to retch. "Nose job?"

"Yup, I gave Aaron a movie-star nose free of charge. You're welcome, buddy." Then to me, she said, "When we got in there we found a deviated septum so we fixed that on our way out."

"Humph," we said in unison, and then all three of us laughed.

One day she walked with us out of the clinic and I saw a name I recognized on a door in hallway. "R. Storey Fenton," I said.

"Uh huh. He's the chief," she replied.

"The same Storey Fenton who's a pilot?"

"Yes, actually, he is."

"No way! He's a friend ... a flying buddy of my father's. He keeps a plane on the ramp beside my father's, in the town where my parents live."

"He also happens to be the guy who invented the technique for the surgery Aaron just had."

Another I-couldn't-make-this-shit-up coincidence. I dug into the medical research at home and found that Michael Cusimano and R. Storey Fenton, both with connections to my father, had been instrumental (pun intended) in surgery being available nearby for my son's uber-rare condition. I would always wonder if we might have ended up in California had these degrees of separation not coalesced in our lives. And I will never doubt the universe again. Turns out that Michael Cusimano was the first surgeon in the world to perform the endoscopic procedure, where a video lens goes into the surgical site along with the instruments. I really wanted to watch one being done. (I'm a geek that way.)

In my research travels I tried to find anything published about how patients coped after surgery, how they felt. I found nothing. Aaron was changed, certainly, and who wouldn't be? But I couldn't name it. Was it more sensitive? Irritable? Teenager-esque? I was treading lightly around him. He unpredictably lost his temper on me a few times — times when I couldn't sluff it off and the sting was such that I needed to get the hell away. He was quick to remind me and those few people he saw that he'd been through hell, most often mentioning being alone in the hospital, having instruments cut into his head, and five days with a catheter.

My kids were those kids that other people always remarked on: even-keeled (except with one another), and expressive. Our parenting style had been geared to meeting their needs, setting expectations, and applying the same standards to ourselves as we demanded of them. Unlike the family I was raised in, calm ruled our home with the boys. "It's not arms and legs" was our mantra. My mother's temper was something I peeked around door frames to check for before entering the room. Her rapier tongue reigned supreme in the family dynamic and was the most significant feature of my childhood. Rick and I were adamant when we first talked about having kids that raised voices and verbal assaults would not be part of our home. And they weren't. Ever.

Because Aaron wasn't enjoying going out, I hosted my immediate family at our house for my sister's birthday. During the meal, my niece Laura asked about the rarity of gigantism and she wanted to know if Aaron would still grow. "He *is* still growing, we think." I would have gone on to answer her other questions, but we got cut off.

"You just can't shut up about it, can you?" Aaron yelled, glaring at me across the table.

I felt like I'd been slapped. Heat seared into me, and I felt the silent vacuum around me as everyone either turned to me awaiting my response or dropped their gaze to their plate. The tears were there before I could chide them into hiding. I pushed my chair back from the table, went to my room, closed and locked the door. I never went back. I don't know how the table was cleared, when the house emptied. I don't know what happened next. I came apart, defeated, crumpled into an emotional, weeping heap in my room.

I explained this to Rick on the phone not too many days later. We spoke often to check in on where the boys would be and when, but also on how Aaron was doing, how he seemed to us.

"Maybe he'll never be the same. Maybe he does hate me," I blubbered.

Then Rick said, "I choose to believe that our kid will be the miracle. I'm just gonna stick my head in the sand until you tell me to get my fucking head out of the sand." How nice for him.

I didn't resemble my former self either. I felt like an onion, and there were no more layers to peel. I identified with that meaty core of the onion that I imagine shudders, shrouding its face while its armour is pulled away. My senses were heightened. The ceramic floor felt so cold. The light from the curtainless windows, once welcoming, now stung my eyes. One night when I was gathering the garbage, a scent made me remember Aaron's in-patient days, and I felt the concrete block weight of worry on my chest again. I'd always been this way. I had this sensorial trigger after spending so much time with Doug, a forty-something man diagnosed with pancreatic cancer about whom I was writing my first book. Moments in palliative care with Doug came back to me vividly with the scent of lavender, the type of body cream I'd applied for him liberally during his bedridden months. My boys' baby and toddler years had always come back to me with the smells of Johnson's baby lotion and powder, or a particular fabric softener that left its impression on freshly folded linens. And then I would be right there again with middle-of-the-night diaper changes, bleary-eyed feedings, but most wonderfully, the tender kisses I planted on their silky cheeks as they fell asleep on my shoulder. That night the association affected me like never before. It sickened me, leaving me feeling grief. My father had begun finishing my basement, building a hockey memorabilia room and guest suite, and when I balled up tape backing, hurling it into a contractor-sized bag, I caught the whiff of latex, plastic, and adhesive. In a olfactory smackdown I was bedside in the hospital in an instant, my boy fighting to breathe through a packed nose after surgery, uncomfortable, dizzy, confused, status unknown. He was the smell of latex to me now. *Will this experience usurp forever the more beautiful memories I have of my sons, of a time when we felt like a family, when I could keep them safe?*

16

PROMISE MAKER

"Why the hell doesn't Dad do anything?"

Justin was pissy, caught somewhere between frustration that I couldn't do something because I had to take his brother to the hospital and worry over my exhaustion. I don't remember what I said no to. I was preoccupied trying to rub some feeling into my numb hands. That had been happening a lot lately — and sometimes I couldn't feel my feet either. I was saying no to almost everything at that point because of scheduling, feeling wrung out, and not wanting to deal with public and social situations. Justin had lost his high-energy, endless-hopper-of-ideas-and-yeses Mom.

I avoided these Dad criticism moments. Rick and I had promised that we wouldn't bash each other. I tried the "Dad *does* help," and its caveat "when I ask" (without adding that I didn't often ask or that Aaron didn't want me to involve Rick). I said, "This has always been my stuff to do for you guys," and "Dad is swamped with work, and my time is more open."

Justin scolded the thick air around him. "Well, we have two parents and you guys actually get along." We were still sitting in the car inside the garage, where the conversation had started as I was pulling in. He wasn't wrong. But this wasn't a conversation I could have with him. "I've got your back, Mom. You don't have to do it alone." My heart swelled. He was such a wonderful young man. Heart on his sleeve, opinions open to the world. "I'll even come to appointments, if Aaron will let me." He got out of the car. I sniffled back tears.

"We both know that isn't gonna happen!" Laughter rescued us again.

The responsibility I had with Aaron's medical path left me with mixed feelings about Rick and his relative lack of involvement. I wasn't upset by it. I felt nothing but empathy. Rick was a doer; I was a worrier, and so much of Aaron's care required anticipating possibilities and what-ifs. As an engineer, Rick avoided undesirable outcomes that he could not will into his control. We coped as we always had. But I missed him terribly, and I couldn't claw my way back now. Asking for help might be seen as manipulative. I'd asked for the separation. This is how it had to be. I had loved him too long and I respected him too much.

I wanted to toss word bombs, of course. On the phone when he would leave me with a placating remark, saying that he couldn't accept that this was happening to our boy, I wanted to tell him to snap the fuck out of it! My upset was around what seemed like disinterest in how the disease worked or could eventually manifest. I sent the links. I'd been sending notes about things I was learning, but he was replying or commenting less and less.

"Why don't you worry more?" I asked him one day. "Why am I worrying so much and you aren't?" It was the best I could manage to confront him around our difference in this.

Tears in his eyes, biting back the quiver in his lip, he said simply, "Because he has you. He has everything he needs."

"Hey, buddy, are you upstairs?" Grunt of teenage-boy acknowledgement audible from somewhere. "Can you come down for a minute?" Nothing. "Aaron, can you puh-lease come down here?"

Beside me, wagging his feathery butterscotch tail, Reef panted with excitement. I held his harness, stopping him from bolting up the two short flights of stairs to find the boys. I wanted this surprise. Aaron wasn't coming. He was still unpredictably grouchy.

"Go get Aaron," I whispered, then I let the joy of hearing Aaron's high-pitched training voice, his loud conversation with Reef, and the general ruckus of giant boy and huge dog collapsing into a tussle on the upstairs carpet fill my heart, freezing a smile on my face for hours.

"I bought him out of slavery," I said later, when Aaron asked me how I'd managed it. Reef had been assessed, was judged to be too anxious and easily distracted for full public-access certification and was offered back to me as an unofficial companion animal (but really as a pet) for a whack of cash I readily paid. There was some guilt assuaging involved for me. As his principal trainer, I'd likely inflicted my own anxiety on him. (You know what they say about how dogs mimic their owners.) I had heard that the separation was difficult for Reef and that the disruption showed in his behaviour. He belonged with us.

I was a walking juxtaposition: Driven by my desire for normalcy for the children, I soothed at any cost, but inside, I was volatile and defensive. I woke in nightmares and was triggered by their horrors through the day. To survive being overcome by fear of Aaron's future, I wouldn't allow myself to think ahead, but by not thinking ahead, I became destructive, laying regrets on my path, which I would never recover from.

Val was still living with us and so was her loveable (but backyard-destroying), goofy bear of a dog, and that had made four dogs in the house. The busyness of the household was a lot for all of us introverts to handle, but I was still surprised when the kids told me they weren't liking it. Aaron said he was feeling judged, like he was on public display. Val was family, I told them, period. But his mood could be dark, and his behaviour occasionally reflected his inner turmoil. The aftermath of diagnosis and surgery was a roller coaster for him. It was making us all living together untenable. But I needed the help to care for my pets, my house, and Justin, when Aaron and I still spent so many hours every day at hospitals in the city. And I'd opened my home to Val after a recent breakup, offering her what I hoped would be stability. Whose comfort would I protect, and how costly would the price be for me? I couldn't win this one.

Like a coward I raised the subject with Val by email while she was at work. It was no shock that I wasn't managing very well. I took great comfort in all the dogs and two queen-sized beds being in my master bedroom. I hadn't really been alone since the move into my house. Her reaction, uncharacteristic of our relationship, was to turn the tables on me. We don't think you're managing all this very well. She'd spoken to Rick, to my family (Kelly, I imagined), and they were considering an intervention. *An intervention? Like with an addict?* You're distant and volatile and emotional. We all need to help you. *Help me? How is anyone supposed to help?*

They couldn't cure my boy, take his fear and discomfort away, assure his future. They had no idea what I'd been through walking the halls of a hospital not knowing if he was dead or alive. But what I wrote back made three points: My son just had brain surgery. I just left my husband. Get your stuff and get the hell out. I didn't recognize myself. Anger, while in my DNA, had never wended its way into my conscience, but self-protection did. I wanted to be alone, under no one's all-assuming gaze. I wanted to be alone to hate myself. I played my part in isolating us and also responded to my inner voice's reminder to stay low, attract no attention, so the predator will just leave. The boys and

I were a three now, a permanent acknowledgement of what had always been a reality with me at home and Rick working so much. But we were so different together now. The boys' relationship was strained. My rapport with each of them was tailored to their unique concerns and anger points. Aaron and I were a comedy duo during hospital trips. I called us Frick and Frack. Justin was getting more annoyed with being left behind at home while his brother and I had what he perceived as *fun* days in the city together. I played whatever song they needed me to. I was pretending around them so much of the time.

"Your boys sure love their mom," Mailie, one of the other hockey moms said at summer camp pick-up one day.

"What makes you say that?" I asked.

"They actually choose to spend time with you. You're always together. At their age, especially, that's amazing.

"I guess so."

"My boys can't get far enough away from me. They tell me that all the time. I'm jealous, Patti."

"Yeah, we're together a lot, but think about why that is." *Be careful what you wish for*, I wanted to say.

"The divorce, you mean?" *Ouch, so that's obviously public chatter.*

"No, it's all the medical stuff. Aaron's stuck going with his mother everywhere and Justin's life gets squeezed into the openings in the calendar. I'm pretty sure they both wish it could be different."

Mailie moved in to hug me. "I'm pretty sure Aaron doesn't see it that way." She had known my boys for eight years. "He knows he wouldn't be as well as he is without you. Remember that, will ya? He's a kid and he can't say it, so I will."

More tears stung my eyes. I didn't want to do it in the arena parking lot. Damn it all.

"You guys actually manage to make it look fun," Mailie said. I smiled back at her and made for the car.

Aaron didn't want to be social and had stopped reaching out to his friends. I noticed that both boys were more contented being at home in the evenings and on weekends than they'd been before, and while that concerned me, it allowed me to stay in too. Hiding was all I wanted to do, and my increasing isolation was justified when the boys were with me.

Despite my conviction to stay alone, the women who were still in my life felt I should be getting out. (Val and I had not patched it up, and she had moved to an apartment in the city.) Dana signed me up on a dating site. Jenny thought I should meet her after work in the city sometime and just go out and be around people again. Jenny, a city girl now, had grown up in the same small town where I lived with the boys. She had the polish, sophistication, and worldliness that I craved, but had no band-width to seek. All *I* wanted was my book and my bed by eight. I hadn't mustered the energy for anything but hospital days in months, and confidence in my appearance had left the building years prior. But I finally gave in to my friend Helen, and met her colleague for dinner one night. Serg was a good-looking, sparkly eyed, intelligent child psychologist. We had dinner at a pub, and while he spoke about being a cigar aficionado and how he spent evenings on the weekends with his single buddies or with the married ones (only if their wives stayed in the kitchen and served up multi-course meals), my mind wandered. Then he asked about my kids. I'm pretty sure I went deep into the medical odyssey, the effects on Aaron, the guilt, maybe even the divorce. He was a psychologist after all. We shook hands and I saw the relief on his face.

I didn't know who to be if it wasn't about the boys, and I wasn't apologetic about it.

At twenty-nine, when I'd learned it was time to become a mother again, I promised a sleeping Aaron, "You'll be one of two soon. You will never have to feel alone." It was reassurance I hadn't always known as a child and my conviction was borne of my sense of loneliness. In my noisy, emotional childhood, there were no boundaries on what should not be said to someone you loved, let alone another sentient being. For the most part I was a surprise to my parents, and nothing more than a nuisance to my siblings. I was no one's preferred companion. Rather like a house chore, I was shuffled and bargained over. "Who's gonna get Patti from piano?" "Who's gonna look after Patti?" "Take your little sister with you." My rejection was assuaged by a cheap multi-tiered bookcase my father ordered me from a catalogue on which I shelved and reshelved my books, first by title, then by author, curating my tiny, precious library. I had a cozy spot in my closet where I would hole up with my things. Out of sight meant out of range of someone's temper and delayed the inevitable announcement that I should be somewhere else, usually in bed. I insisted it would feel different for my boys. I wanted them to know that the celebration they were at birth had never ended for me. And they do. In fact, they love to tease me about being weepy at their accomplishments or when they hug me or when they walk in the door.

One Saturday evening when Aaron dozed off, a big, sloppy pile of teenager on the couch, all jeans and hoodie and ball cap, a death-grip on the clicker, I had a rare chance to watch him sleeping. The profile was a stretched, puffed-up extension of his youthful one. I could still see his toddler face in the shadows, lying with his hands flung above his head. I had seen that nose, pooked-out mouth (Hall family lingo for lips on a little one that look like an aesthetician Lubridermed them), and tiny chin in the ultrasound before he relocated himself outside of me. Later, when he was eight, I saw that profile in the brightness cast by his plastic dolphin nightlight in the room that was painted like an ocean because he wanted his room to be "like another world, Mama, like the sky."

Standing bedside, I had promised to be fair and good and kind. I said it out loud as I watched them sleep, always clear on my wishes for the kind of mother I would be, more so for the mother I would *not* be. There were hurdles, and I failed miserably many times. I'd set the bar pretty high. The challenges posed by a two-year-old alone ensured I would waver, if nothing else. But even unrelenting love and our permanent ties could not prepare us for the disaster as great as chronic illness. It could have broken us. Maybe it was supposed to. Maybe it still would.

But I had promised him. *Did he get what I promised? What would he say? Did he get the mother he deserved?*

By July's end, while the boys savoured the lazy days, Justin doing some sports camps and Aaron perfecting channel surfing from the couch, I was trying to remember what my life had been like six months before — before the separation, the move, the diagnosis ... What the hell had I planned to do next? Where was that book I'd been writing and how was I going to get focused on growing my career?

This is what we were talking about one evening, as Dana, Jenny, and I were sipping wine and snacking. And then my cell-phone rang. Dr. Schwinn was the endocrinologist Aaron had seen prior to surgery. I cringed a little. Aaron had never been comfortable with her. (And that's putting it mildly.) She was one of the primary physicians who had not established some rapport with him, awkwardly calling him "son," speaking over him (not easy to do when he was standing up) and past him, wanting answers only from me. I'd even seen her tilt her head in the isn't-he-cute posture that people use around annoying toddlers. Perhaps Dr. Schwinn was just another reality of having a teenager in an adult environment, but I simply expected better. Period. Aaron had asked me to get him another endocrinologist many times, but I knew the efficacy of having a consulting endocrinologist with privileges at the hospital where his neurosurgical team lived far outweighed this personality conflict. I knew the smart way to play this medical game, and I was a coward, not wanting to lose medical support I'd despaired to find. Aaron's wishes were something I could manage so long as the doctor was not downright rude to him or incompetent.

"Hi, Mrs. Hall. I'm looking at your son's results and it looks like he's incurable."

And there it was. The iceberg had appeared out of the dim, and I was Frederick Fleet, the Titanic's night lookout, calling, "Iceberg, right ahead!"

Easy for you to fucking say. I might have actually said that. She'd be great to have as the lead doctor in a crisis. I could imagine her yelling through a megaphone, "Sorry folks, but you're all gonna die today."

If there was a conversation after that, I couldn't have contributed much. I know that I got off the phone as quickly as possible because I'd decided I'd never take Aaron back to her anyway.

I went to the washroom as soon as I put the phone down and looked at myself in the mirror. That doctor left no space for faith or denial. *It looks like he's incurable.* There it was, my boy's iceberg. After all this. My kid wouldn't be getting the clean bill, wouldn't be receiving the reward of security. For months I had been gritting and grinding, chugging and chomping at tasks I would never have undertaken for myself. And yet a cure was not coming. The surgery had made some improvement to his endocrine levels, but it had failed to lower his growth hormone to a normal range. The residual tumour would carve a path in the rest of Aaron's life, determining his degree of safety, influencing his confidence and state of mind, and predicting his quality of life. I was no match for it.

The phone call had forged into coal the dust of despair I'd been unable to digest for months. When I woke on Sunday morning, the silence was profound. My first breath happened and then I listened for the sound of the boys in the house, and that day there was nothing. The dogs were there but not moving. I was alone.

A band of anxiety tightened around my belly. My legs felt like lead and my eyes hurt to be open, so I pulled the pillow over my head. I could not will myself to get up or fidget my body into a comfortable position. I stayed contorted under the pile of blankets and sobbed.

When I forced myself up that evening because the boys were coming home from their weekend at Rick's, I saw clumps of hair on the pillow.

I called the therapist I'd begun to see in the lead up to the separation from Rick, and left her a message saying I was feeling worse than ever before, I was down twenty pounds, couldn't keep food down even when I could stand to eat, and I couldn't stop crying. At our next appointment, she started in with the self-care platitudes, but my panic cut her off. I needed her to know that I was drowning. I told her about the numbness in my hands and feet, joint pain, shortness of breath, disorientation, tightness in my chest, falling asleep while driving, nausea, painful urination, chronic diarrhea. I was having recurring nightmares of racing toward something but never arriving because tragedy interrupted. I was losing track of time and the date, and my short-term memory was lapsing. I had to write everything down on Post-its. I felt afraid all the time, to the point of paranoia. I had the shakes, was weak in the knees, and I was tripping a lot. I admitted how alone I felt, how abandoned. And I wouldn't let anyone help me because I didn't want them to see what I mess I was.

"You may have to let them help you," she said. I repressed my ire. I was so sick of hearing that I needed help. *I'm at the damn therapist, aren't I?*

"Whaddya mean?"

"I think you're going to need to say yes to some support." Depression was well known to me. I'd descended into it for a few dark months fifteen years before, weighed down by apathy, physical weakness, back and joint pain, light sensitivity, and nausea that was debilitating. And I'd needed help to care for the kids and my pets because Rick travelled about a third of the year in our first decade together. But I'd been rationalizing and denying for months and I hadn't acknowledged that I was in real trouble, beyond anything I'd been through before.

"It's a depressive episode, isn't it? I'm slipping into the pit again."

There is a place this side of hysteria where I'd hovered, and I was paying the price now. Rather than rant it somewhere safe, I buried it. *No one can really understand what I'm going through*, I faultily reasoned, and I hid my lonely embittered mood behind "I'm doing okay" and "No, I don't need anything." I was on a collision course with my own wellness. I wasn't going to right myself this time. I was going down. Abandon ship. I heard seven short horn blasts and a long-sustained wail that may have been coming from me.

17

PATIENT

When the boys were with me, I did anything I could to manage, buoying myself up with strong coffee, cooking their favourite potato chowder and mac and cheese, mindlessly knitting yet another lap blanket while they watched television. I couldn't let them see me crumbling. I didn't want them feeling responsible for me. I faked it.

Medication had been effective for me before, and when my doctor suggested an increase, I acquiesced. I was in no position to question her. It was the only way I could keep up the facade, like wearing a tensor bandage on my brain. There was another impetus for the pretense. I didn't want them taking the news of "Mom cries all the time" or "Mom doesn't even get out of her pyjamas when she drives us to school" back to their dad. In the months when we were negotiating our separation agreement, I'd seen notes once when Rick's day planner lay open by the telephone. "Depression, custody, incapacity." Rick was doing his homework.

So I lived two lives. When the boys were with Rick on alternate weekends, I holed up in my room under the covers, sleeping for twelve-hour stretches and getting up only to feed the dogs or let them out, ensuring that two days later when I heard the car pull into the driveway, I could bolt out of bed and assume the familiar posture of stirring a huge pot of Sunday dinner on the stove. Medication helped to quiet the self-deprecating thoughts and the rumination over my mistakes, and quell the paralyzing fears I now had when I thought of the months ahead — managing life, house, responsibilities, and finances without a partner.

I reached out to my sister, who had seen some glimpses of the foreboding lethargy, despair, and compulsive weeping that occupied my time without the boys, just to tell her I was really feeling rough, and then regretted it immediately. Kelly's response would be the best she could do, suggestions about getting out, questions about seeing my doctor, reminders that I could get through it because I was the strongest person she knew. I could hear nothing, do nothing. I waded through, hour by hour, from complete hopelessness to accepting this might be my new normal.

And I desperately wanted faith. I wanted the relief of laying myself at the feet of a God that would heal Aaron, bring Justin the mother he needed back, and thereby heal us all. I wanted someone I could offer my sacrifice to. Take me, save him. I saw myself bargaining, the way that cancer sufferers did in Kübler-Ross's initial work about the five stages of grief.

The most shameful part, which manifested and bloomed exponentially in the alone hours, was that I wanted to flee, abdicate, yes, take off. If I was not doing it well enough, I wanted to stop trying. I wanted someone else to do it. My anxiety had maxed out. Everything I'd been doing still wasn't enough. I didn't want to make decisions about the rest of his life. I didn't want to sit in rooms violating his dignity by talking about his puberty and whether we might supplement him with testosterone. I didn't want that power. I didn't want to be the one breaking more bad news to him, inflicting course-altering diversions on his life.

I didn't want to be Mom anymore.

But if not me, then who? Aaron would not make decisions. And he wouldn't allow his Dad to be any more involved. These boys were why I was on the planet, and I needed to survive, if not rise. So, tormented by the winless situation, I just gave in to sleep, hoping one day I would wake up feeling like I could cope.

The weeks and months that followed were a haze of heady fog. I searched for a reason to get up (them), to stay up (get them to school), and to leave my bed in the afternoon (school was over). Muscle tension and pain like I'd never known before had enveloped my body. My legs and arms lost circulation as I drove. I strained against the pain of twisting to step out of my vehicle and I struggled to straighten when I got up from the table. *So this is where the stress has been hiding,* I thought. When I could think at all.

One day I was unable to stop crying. My mother, on her weekly check-in phone call, simply said, "I'm coming over" and then to my shock she showed up.

"You get right into bed," she said, pulling the covers up to my neck. "This might take months but you are going to survive. You have to survive." She awkwardly pulled the antique cane-seated chair out from under the schoolhouse desk that sat decoratively under my bedroom window, sat down, and watched me sleep for hours.

This was the saddest moment of my life. I had never known her help except in Aaron's early weeks of life, and she had never come to me unasked.

"You need to see your doctor," my mother said when I woke, in her typical harsh tone.

"I do. I have. I'm at a high dose of my antidepressants." I was chilled yet sweating, eyes pinched against the light, scratching at the cracked hive-like welts on my arms and neck.

My mother was a self-professed clinical expert on all things cancer, terminal disease, palliative care, and shit she had seen working in the ER and surgical departments of the local hospital where we grew up. But mental health was the domain of the old wives' tale with her. Depression wore many euphemisms in her medical dictionary, like "the blues" and "the dumps." It had never been afforded a modicum of scientific seriousness by her. Yet that day, she told me that she'd been on a low-dose antidepressant herself for twenty years. It was like someone lifted the window blind to peer out, and the light cracked in. Of course that statement was followed by the usual disclaimers that I'd heard from everyone who'd taken meds for depression or anxiety, all of them shamed into feeling like idiots or addicts or both for trying medication with the hope of easing their own suffering and returning to life: "It's just a little bit," "The doctor says it's not much," "I can stop taking it anytime," "I did my research and there are no known side effects," etc. She'd "gone down" before too, like when I was an infant and my colic went six weeks straight and the family physician medicated her rather than me. I was glad she was there, even though I was repressing the thoughts of who she might tell or how she might throw her kindness back in my face in the future. Just when I thought her empathy would extend to understanding and mark a breakthrough for our relationship, she said, "There now, you've had a good sleep. I'm going home and I'll call you tomorrow." I imagined an orchestral flourish and her superhero cape flipped over her shoulder as she left my room. *My work here is done.*

When I was with the boys, I had to be *on*, and so I was.

"I've got one, Mom," Aaron said. "*Life is short; I'm not.*"

"Yup, that's a good one," I said. I'd told Aaron about Sandy Allen, the tallest living woman in the world until 2008, according to Guinness. When she spoke to schoolchildren (from her wheelchair in later years) she always wore a T-shirt with a funny saying on it, like "How'd you get so short?" or "I'm with shorty." Making up slogans had become one of our sources of amusement.

They got more rudely sarcastic as time went on. I told Aaron that Sandy Allen had died the year before his diagnosis. He didn't ask the cause or her age, and I don't know if he looked it up himself when he was alone. I wasn't sure if he wondered what his own life would be like in the years ahead.

But one thing we'd discussed was his taking medication. Before we decided to find a new endocrinologist, Dr. Schwinn had told us that Aaron would have to accept that he may need medication for the rest of his life. The tumour suppressant, Sandostatin, could cost close to $100,000 a year depending on dosage. She said it like it was a daily aspirin. Why use a sledgehammer when a feather duster will do? I'd looked up this drug and knew its carcinogenic effects were being researched. I also knew it was considered the best option to keep a tumour remnant like Aaron's in check, if anything could. I still needed to find another endocrinologist to manage Aaron's care. One with more experience and some bedside manner. And it would be a bonus if my kid didn't turn into a raging menace in that doctor's presence!

I went back to the source of all knowledge in my life — my hairdresser, Vicki. It should have been funny that in my search for a world expert on this uber-rare endocrine disorder, the key resource was my sassy, brilliant hairstylist, the one I pelted with profanity when she diagnosed my kid from a school picture. This woman, who might have been either a criminal mastermind or the lead brain in a tech startup or both (and she can deal with naturally curly hair too, which by anyone's standards makes her a rock star), dropped the name of the endocrinologist Aaron needed into the palm of my waiting hand, between the trim and the blow dry. I asked Dr. Kirsch to write to Dr. Shereen Ezzat and she kindly sent a note: "GH levels high again. Parents requesting your expertise for further management choices."

The soft-spoken, slight man with a handshake that felt like a kid-leather glove, Dr. Ezzat was the first person who sounded thoroughly versed in all aspects of the disease treatment, and crucial for me, he believed Aaron's age was an asset, not a liability. Finally, an expert. I didn't dare allow myself to consider how getting to Ezzat earlier might have altered treatment options or outcomes. That water needed to stay under the bridge. We had the doctor now, but that only meant an additional crew member. We still had no map. Treatment would be lifelong, but what would be best? What were the statistics, the risks, and the range of outcomes? I did what writers do. I turned again to the internet, something I'd been avoiding or perhaps just hadn't had the energy to look at since Aaron's surgery. There were going to be more choices to make. There wasn't going to be time to settle into the reassuring calm. Aaron was still very much in the acute phase of his disease. I harnessed all the energy I had and directed it at the problem, diving into some research, my favourite avoidance strategy. I was not willing to point my attention to my own mental state.

I found some short-lived consolation — it was common for the disease to go undiagnosed for ten years. I also saw the symptom list again, honing in on the ones that persisted in Aaron, like hypertension, sleep apnea, hyperhidrosis, and inflammation in the weight-bearing joints. I was reminded that the situation is almost always more extreme and the effects more severe in pituitary gigantism than in acromegaly because the discovery of the tumour occurred prior to growth stopping.

But my interest was piqued by how long the disease had been known (no one seemed to agree because medical science and mythology were at odds with one another). Very little progress had been made in a century or more. Since the work by Dr. Pierre Marie in the 1880s and Maximilian Sternberg's *Acromegaly* of 1899, there were fewer than a dozen substantive publications on acromegaly or gigantism. I read case studies, descriptions, verbatim reports of sufferers before the turn of the last century. It was fascinating. I felt embers, if not a familiar fire in my belly. I wanted to know everything. And I couldn't stop reading. *Could this be my thing? Is this what will drag me kicking and screaming out of the pit?*

"Another appointment with no good news. We *never* get good news." Aaron pushed the elevator button and led us to the hospital food court. A few minutes later he looked at me across his plate of food. "I'm learning to keep this in a box," he said.

"A box?"

"Yeah, like, I only think about it when we're here or I'm having a needle or an MRI; otherwise I put all of this in a box."

Aaron considered himself pre-disasterized; he'd seen the worst in his estimation, so he calibrated inversely. He measured bad news as the constant and good news as the oddity. He compartmentalized, a really sophisticated way to deal with trauma, and it broke my heart.

"Well, at least today wasn't *bad* news," he said.

Did he hear the same thing I did? We'd been told that his IGF-1 was still higher than normal. Things were not improving.

"What would bad news have been then, buddy?"

He thought for a moment. "Good question. Guess I don't know the answer to that. For that matter, what the hell would good news be? We know I'm not getting better."

I wouldn't lie to him. I kept eating.

It was my job to bear the news, digest the shocks, and soften the blows. He had concluded this one on his own.

One day I flipped a stack of mail over and saw an envelope addressed to Aaron, with the blue printed return address of the hospital network. Without much thought, expecting a confirmation of an MRI or blood-testing appointment, I ripped it open. It was an appointment booking, but the doctor's name wasn't one I knew, and it was at a hospital we'd never been to. Dr. Ezzat's efficient assistant Anna had attached a note telling me it was just a copy to confirm the appointment. Why had Dr. Ezzat referred Aaron to someone else?

He'd had surgery less than one year before. Was Aaron's health devolving so rapidly or so significantly that another surgery was warranted? *Is this an emergency? Is Aaron sicker than I've been told?* I ran as fast as I could to grab my phone.

I'm not proud of the message I left the specialist that day. In short, I lost it. I resorted to email next and let Dr. Ezzat's assistant know that there is a reason why patients are informed of the progress of their health, their diagnosis, or the need for referrals. I went on about the right to know, to not be the last to know, and how in our case especially, I had a teenage kid to break the news to. *Why the hell am I finding out that my kid is sicker than I thought in a piece of mail?*

Thoughtless experiences were innumerable in those months; they are a reality for anyone who finds themself in the medical system and they are spirit-breaking. I remember a neurosurgeon looking me in the eye, telling me that he was disappointed to say that *my* results showed there was no improvement in *my* tumour. He had picked up the wrong chart and come looking for a female. There was the time when Aaron attended an endocrine appointment by himself and was told that his levels were increasing (they had been downtrending for a long time), his growth-hormone level had doubled since his appointment three months earlier, and someone would call him about his next appointment. After he texted me this, I checked the blood results on the internet patient portal and saw that the number Aaron had been given was for another blood result entirely. Yet — and this is essential — as often as we scoffed at long wait times and administrative mistakes, we always realized that if we had time to be ticked off, Aaron's health must be improving. In moments of true crisis, we always felt responded to. We were so damned grateful and that got us through times when it would have been easy to be annoyed.

18

CELLMATE

He's still here. He's still here. I reached over tentatively to squeeze
Rick's forearm. He looked down at my grip on him and then met
my eyes, as wet with tears as his were, and we smiled knowingly to
one another. "He did it," Rick whispered, lip quivering. We were all
still here, still able to do this together. And we had more to celebrate
than every other family in that crowded high-school gymnasium.

I was sure we were prouder than most parents when Aaron
walked across the stage at graduation. It wasn't the Ontario
Scholar or the extra credit for doing four years of French, and it
wasn't the principal announcing he'd be going to university. For
us, it was that Aaron was here to see this day, to walk unaided and
without pain across this stage (in his extra-long gown), with a
tassel dangling annoyingly in his face like everyone else. He was
as well as we could hope. Justin stood on a chair between us to
see his brother, and after I told him to get down, he used me to
lean on as he jumped, first slipping his arm across my shoulders.
Then he said into my ear, "You didn't think he'd make it here
did you, Mom?"

That wasn't exactly it, but I gave Justin a one-armed hug and said, "He might not have, Jay." Rituals interrupt and punctuate every day, pulling our attention above the noise, the scuttlebutt of to-do's, the hurrying up, the getting it all done. Aaron's graduation was a complex milestone, a figurative line in the sand — both a finishing line and a starting line. He could be anything he wanted now, Rick and I told him in the car driving to the ceremony. "You get to make all the choices now," Rick said. Aaron had crossed this line, ascended to this terrace on the climb to adulthood, but I still quailed when I thought of his future. Could he step in now to become his own advocate, call the shots, manage his medical life? Was he ready to make those choices, as well as the ones about school and career, cars and girlfriends?

I'd had two years of intense access, watching Aaron adapt, morph, mature, and grow into himself (pun intended). It had been like holding a leaf up to a brightly lit window and seeing the intricate system of circulation that fed its growth. We'd been wedged into exam rooms, elevators, and blood labs, and we'd altered simultaneously in situ, like trees that intertwine because of proximity while seeking their space in the sun. We laughed to manage. Our laughter was our management technique, our serum for survival.

Hospital hijinks and not-always-classy waiting-room behaviour was one of our greatest sources of levity. While other waiters fingered sheets of paper or stared at the meaningless mission statements and handwritten signage plastered randomly on the walls, we were those two people in giggle fits, covering our smirks, whispering to one another. Sometimes it would be jokes and videos on our phones, but I'm not proud to say it was often about the odd behaviour of folks in the hospital. Our people-watching was always tempered with sympathy because we'd been there. We might snicker in lobbies, but we were polite, quiet, and respectful when we moved up floors to the inner sanctum of departments where folks just like us were getting their own life-altering bad news. We made up stories about the people seated with us. Who were they to each other? What were they here for? Who was the patient and who was the sidekick?

"No way, Mom. You're wrong. She is waaay too old to be his sister. She has to be the mother or the *grand*mother. She is old, Mom!" *Brat.*

"Aaron, that woman is younger than I am. I'm forty-five years old."

"Yeah, like I said, *ancient*."

"Bad child."

"Yeah, but I'm your favourite."

"You *are* my favourite oldest son, yes."

Sometimes, but only sometimes, we'd talk about what was going to happen that day. There were a couple of points of discomfort — my discomfort — that I always wished I could get Aaron to handle differently. (He had not yet become his own decision-maker and every chance he could, he continued to defer to me.) Testosterone was one of these awkward points for me. We never spoke about it, because I could never raise it with him without him shutting me down, yet it was part of every endocrine checkup he had. And I wasn't going to embarrass my son by asking him for details about puberty.

At one appointment a twentysomething, pale, svelte French doctor was the endocrine specialist who spoke with us before Ezzat (he was a one word entity to us now, like Cusimano) came in. She was incredibly competent. I felt sorry for her because Aaron could be blunt and unyielding with his mildly annoyed attitude when answering the litany of questions he had responded to hundreds of times. Struggling with English, she followed the same routine as every other clinician. With Aaron seated up on the examining table, she asked about his back and joint pain, measured his fingers, checked his vision, confirmed his pulse, and was so surprised by his blood pressure she did it twice. We sniggered.

"Yes, that's about Aaron-normal, don't worry," I said. When Aaron came back to the chair beside me, she asked about his sleep, energy level, muscle mass, and about lumps and polyps and inevitably, "Have you reached sexual maturity?"

"How would I know? I have nothing to compare it to." Then, dead air. Radio silence.

This was a typical office visit. No one was ever either concerned enough or willing enough to violate his privacy and ask more probing questions. That would be a sweet story if puberty was not so important to his quality of life in the future. I knew that testosterone was often prescribed for people with pituitary disorders to keep them feeling energetic and to sustain their libido. But I also remembered that one of the doctors had told Aaron once that as a steroid, the effects of testosterone on the remnant tumour were unknown. Aaron had been clear. If there was any chance that taking testosterone would prompt his tumour to grow — no thank you.

Sometimes I pushed harder than others. Sooner or later he would want to advocate for himself, I was certain. At another appointment a thirtysomething round-faced endocrine intern noticed Aaron's birthdate and said bluntly, "Oh, you're eighteen now. We can ask your mother to wait outside while we talk, then."

I nodded and stood up, picking up the medical binder and my bag from the floor, happy to exit. My inside voice was giving a *woo-hoo!*

"She's not leaving," Aaron said. "If she leaves, I'm going too. She's the only one that knows what's going on with me. She needs to stay."

"It's okay, buddy, you've got this."

"No, Mom. This is how we do this. I don't care if I'm eighteen. Let's just do it like we always have."

I sat. The doctor said something about Aaron needing to sign a form allowing me access to his medical information.

"I'll sign whatever." In his own way, he was running things. I guess I wanted to be done. Maybe I'd been hoping his age would give me an exit strategy. It wasn't that I didn't want to know what was happening with his health, I wanted him to feel capable. And I was also a coward. I knew at some point he would ask me questions I didn't want to answer. I walked on eggshells at each appointment, wondering what question might bubble to the surface. I wanted to be his sidekick, the clown to help him manage the anxiety, and only in my nightmares did I try to prepare for the questions I never wanted him to ask, like *Am I going to die, Mom? Can I be a father? Will I have to use a walker someday?*

After I'd lost my calm when the letter referring Aaron to another neurosurgeon had surprised me, I arranged to have a phone call with Dr. Ezzat, and I saw that his assistant unfortunately didn't know me for my humour but for something else when she asked me to not shoot the messenger. (So much for my rule about being calm and kind with assistants.) My ranting phone message and follow-up email had evidently left an impression. Now I was that mother I'd never wanted to be. The temperamental, emotional, outbursting one; the high-maintenance one. I was told to answer a blocked number at a certain time on a Friday. Dr. Ezzat was there when I picked up. I was prepared to meet with arrogance and perhaps be reminded that I was out of line, but instead he opened by saying no one had intended for the shock I felt. Then we had a frank discussion about Aaron's health. He said some things on that call that stuck with me for years after. I never respected a physician more than when, in his frankness, he said that when his team first saw Aaron their goal was something like, "We just want to get this kid to thirty." I asked the questions I could never ask in front of my son, unembarrassed by the cracking of my voice, the rattling caused by a lump in my throat. "What will he die of?" He told me that pressure on Aaron's musculoskeletal system would be his greatest challenge, and we would need to closely watch his circulation and the long-term effects of the medication, as well as possible gastrointestinal issues. He could even develop diabetes. We agreed on how *together* we would support Aaron through the time ahead. Dr. Ezzat said he wanted us to be good cop, bad cop. "I'll be hope, and you be the truth," Dr. Ezzat said. He wanted Aaron to expect positive outcomes, and to keep up his willingness to adjust medication and repeat procedures.

Dr. Ezzat explained that the Sandostatin injection, which Aaron received every three weeks, had achieved its maximum effectiveness for now, and he told me that the Tumour Review Board, a collection of experts in many disciplines from three hospitals, which met regularly to review all cases for patients with pituitary tumours, had decided that Aaron should have a consult with Dr. Fred Gentili.

The worst of the depressive months were behind me, but I was very aware that a dose of reality about Aaron's prognosis had triggered me once and the same could again. But something was different this time — I didn't feel like I was going to have to support Aaron myself.

Writers write. It was what I knew to do. Writing may have saved me in the most unconventional of ways — by making my receding from the medical and all things giant impossible, permanently making me live in the face of this new drop-in unannounced visitor who we could never ask to leave. The manuscript about companioning Doug in his final months with pancreatic cancer was pressed lovingly into a box on the corner of my writing desk, and I knew it needed to wait until I was clear about its trajectory. A promise delayed was not a promise broken.

I'd journalled daily during my depressive months. Some of the pieces found their way to my blog, Put Simply. But now what was coming out was narrative — longer stories, memories, and reflections on what it felt like to be bedside with Aaron, fearing for his life, fearing everything. What would I do with what was pouring out of me now, two years after his diagnosis? Could my role as a bedside companion, first for Doug and now for Aaron, guide my writing? Could this be a book? There hadn't been time to plan my next career steps, when being newly separated, single parenting, and Aaron's diagnosis all coincided. *I'm a sidekick*, I thought. *I'll write about that some more.*

I looked online for support groups, information sites, charities. There was almost nothing for acromegaly and certainly zero for gigantism.

"Maybe we should found our own," I suggested to Aaron. We even came up with a name: Pituitary Matters. I did find a group called Acromegaly Community and its founder, Wayne Brown, who guided me to a couple of posts by caregivers — partners, parents, and family members who were the second pair of ears for their loved one. I got into a couple of email exchanges with a few people. A woman called Tina, the partner of a man recently diagnosed with a pituitary tumour in England, told me that there was work being done in London around a genetic explanation for the disease. In all my time on the web, I'd only seen open-ended statements about work being done toward a genetic connection. We had no idea where the disease came from, and there hadn't been conclusive genetic discoveries in 2009. I followed the link Tina offered to me, and on the research page for the Familial Isolated Pituitary Adenoma (FIPA) patients, a charity page was set up for families of people with gigantism and acromegaly who were involved in research taking place in the Department of Endocrinology at St. Bartholomew's Hospital in London. I dropped a few sentences into the contact field. Very little was posted at that point, just a few sentences and a contact link really, but there was something that struck me:

Researchers believe that some 5 percent of tumours might have a genetic explanation.

My cellphone rang on a Sunday night amid the melee of getting Justin out the door to hockey, feeding dogs, boiling pasta, responding to emails, and listening to Aaron talk me through his latest university criminology essay. I answered even though the number looked like a bizarre string of digits with no brackets or hyphens for area codes.

Rather than emailing me back, Dr. Marta Korbonits was calling to explain our options for becoming involved in her work, and to answer any questions I might have about my son. I talked her through the family tree on both sides. I put her on speaker because I needed to take notes, retrieve file folders of information, and flip through Aaron's medical binder. I was nervous, partly because of the importance of this potential connection and my nonclinical background, but also because Aaron hadn't wandered away yet; instead he stayed seated at the kitchen table, hearing it all.

Rock, meet hard place.

The conversation moved quickly through his diagnosis, surgeries, medication, and the names of every member of his medical team. She knew Ezzat and said that us having access to him was a very good thing for Aaron's future. She took me back to all of Aaron's symptoms, his gait, his huge appetite, his constant sweating. She asked about everyone's height in our family and wanted to know levels of Aaron's growth hormone, cortisol, testosterone, and thyroid. Some of her questions seemed so unconnected, but I'd learned by now to listen and respond rather than second-guess these few specialists who knew about co-morbidities and rare combinations of symptoms.

Aaron looked up at me, his eyes widening when the thickly accented Ukrainian-born doctor said, "We need people to understand that giants die in their twenties. We need there to be no more giants." Defensiveness rose within me. *But my son is a giant. And he's here. What about him?*

I quickly shifted back to her point. She meant prevention. If the genetic cause could be found, it could be screened for. I saw what she meant, but it felt so blunt. Of course, medical research is premised on eliminating occurrence; the goal is that there would be no more people with a certain disease. But those still living with it must endure it.

What the hell am I going to say when I put the phone down?

I went for humour and failed. "So, you may be genetically linked to the Irish Giant. *Now* do you believe that we were Irish way back before we were Canadian?" My kids never believed that my passion for all things Celtic was validated by my family history, something now quite relevant. We were as much Irish as we were Scottish, and in one phone call, that heritage had become very important. Aaron wasn't reactive. He was no more interested in me bringing up the Celtic-lineage point than he was in the person on the phone.

Dr. Korbonits was the lead researcher in the discovery of AIP (aryl hydrocarbon receptor–interacting protein) gene mutation, announced to the medical world in the *New England Journal of Medicine* in January 2011. Korbonits's discovery proved family lore, stories passed down generations in County Derry and County Tyrone in Northern Ireland. People there said that Charles Byrne, the famous Irish Giant, who stood seven feet seven inches, was born near where some Irish individuals living with gigantism reside now. In a DNA sample taken from Charles Byrne's preserved skeleton (on display in the Hunterian Museum in London), Korbonits's team confirmed that the mutation present in one of those Irish individuals with gigantism, Brendan Holland, matched that of Byrne. The discovery could mean the medical ability to prevent more people being born with gigantism, or as she said it to me, it could prevent more giants.

But something else had me running to my room that night, pulling the pillow over my head and screaming into the mattress. As if on pulleys, and Korbonits the cosmic set changer, the beachhead rose in front of me. Of the sixteen members of the family we had discussed, the person at highest risk of having gigantism was Justin.

There was the foghorn's mournful tone. We've run aground, crew. Bail like hell, we've run aground. There *was* a new unthinkable creeping its way on deck. I didn't recognize its face, because I'd never even contemplated its existence. The one thing worse than the unthinkable — my son being diagnosed with an incurable, stigma-inviting, pain-inducing, life-limiting uber-rare disease — was the possibility that *both* my sons could be targeted by it. I'd found the dragons, which ancient navigators feared on uncharted areas of the maps. They had my children in their slobbery mouths, flames tickling my boys' heels.

Later it worsened still, as I mentally reviewed the call's outcome ... that she would map our family and tell me who else was at highest risk. *What about my nieces, the cousins on Rick's side, everyone in both of our extended families? And what about us, me and Rick? Could it be brewing in us? Is my nose getting wider now? Didn't I just find my favourite running shoes were getting tight?*

"I suggest strongly that you have Aaron's brother tested," she'd said. She also told me about two teenage patients she had in London right now, brothers with gigantism. She offered to connect me with them.

Dr. Korbonits wanted to speak to Rick's Uncle Grant herself. When I called to get his permission to share his contact information, Grant told me he had a secreting pituitary tumour removed in Missouri in the 1980s, after he experienced loss of vision. He didn't remember a diagnosis, just the tumour. He knew what medications he was still taking, but not what the imbalance was. I left this to Dr. Korbonits to puzzle out. Not long after, she emailed me a family map and assigned us numbers and codes for her study data sets.

I told Rick it was his call about who to tell. His family didn't keep in contact with me after the separation. I offered to have them call me if they were concerned or wanted to know what to look for. I don't know what he did with the information.

Everyone has heard something of giants, whether in folklore, mythology, or children's literature. There have been legends of Celtic giants for centuries, offered as the explanation behind things like Giant's Causeway and the lore of Brian Boru. I'd become fascinated with how the medical reality had crossed into the world of story, myth, and legend. And it came up almost daily when I responded to people staring at us or pointing or asking questions.

"How'd he get so tall?" Mr. Curious would ask.

"He's a giant," I'd answer. Baffled look on Mr. Curious's face. "He suuure is!" (Curious would then self-consciously laugh at his own funny.)

"No, he's a real giant. He has the disease called gigantism." Sometimes Mr. Curious would reel in my boring response and walk away, still staring, but most times he probed further. "Like André the Giant?" or "Like Jack and the Beanstalk?" or "Doesn't Tony Robbins (or the guy who played Lurch or Yao Ming or Jaws from the Bond movie) have that?"

"Yup." And we'd move on down the street, out of the restaurant, into a store, back into our privacy.

But I was a researcher who was also a mother. I couldn't read *Jack the Giant Killer* without being offended. I was cracked open knowing that the bad rap giants got in literature would follow my son all of his days, him and every person of extreme height or size. I started casually collecting via internet download, gleaning from volumes in dusty used bookstores, and purchasing from rare online stores. What continued to intrigue me and to raise my maternal protective dander was that the features of the storied giants, right back to Goliath in the Bible, were medically accurate. But they became monstrous in folkloric depictions. The actual symptomology of people with gigantism, the thick tongue, frontal bossing, poor eyesight, clumsiness, and awkward gait were not storybook features to me, they were real for people with gigantism and acromegaly. This is the not the place to debate societal norms of beauty or to challenge stigmas and presumptions our society has around size. I'll leave that to another book. But just glance at art, film, and the internet and you'll see what marketers use to sell products and services to all of us — grace and lightness. People pray for angels. People fear giants. This disease and societal stupidity had landed my darling in the waters of the monstrous. And I could either turn my gaze away or jump in. If Aaron couldn't avoid it, I would not.

But that wasn't my decision right away. I took too long arranging for blood samples to be sent to the UK for the Irish gene study. It was a pain to organize, but we were two years into this journey and I really liked the calm. I liked not having to go to as many appointments or contemplate how Aaron might regress again. He was stable, or as stable as possible, thanks to the Sandostatin shots he received from Kamilah, the same nurse that had been with us for two years now. Upon hearing that Aaron had begun his university courses, Dr. Ezzat had said, "You have some leeway right now. Go be normal."

I didn't want to interrupt it, not even with a blood test. I wanted to hide my head in a thousand-page historical romance. Round Two had taken an even more dramatic turn — all this could happen to Justin — and I couldn't face it. It took weeks to get Justin checked and more weeks still to arrange with a private medical lab to take blood from Rick, Aaron, and me and ship it to England for the study. Our lives hung in the balance, but only if I thought about it. So I played in the land of denial for a while and absorbed myself in studying the history and geography of giants. And like Aaron, I put into a box the voodoo doll that could take me down once again.

As the lab techs drew our blood, the three of us in a small cubicle, all of us thinking the same what-ifs, dreading a fresh impetus that would toss us into the drink again, Aaron said, "It is what it is." Rick and I smiled at him while in tandem we held our arms out for the bloodletting. "You know, I've been thinking about the tumour," Aaron said. Rick and I instinctively looked at each other, asking silently if the other knew what was coming.

"Oh, yeah? What about it?" Rick said.

"I have to give the tough little bastard credit," he said, smiling. "We're hitting it with everything we've got and still it's holding on. It's almost impressive."

19

WISH SEEKER

"There must be something that Aaron would like. Something that would give him a lift or make the drag of the appointments or getting poked with needles go away for a while ..." My friend Calvin had been a volunteer with the Starlight Wish Foundation.

"Nothing I can think of," I said.

"I mean something bigger than you and Rick could get for him," Calvin said. "I mean trips, a lifetime supply of Cheezies, tickets to a game, a fancy bike, something like that."

I shook my head.

"Well, he would qualify for a wish, I'm sure," Calvin said.

The Starlight warehouse was like the best toy store I'd ever been in. It was heartwarming to see how generously companies donated. Long rows of bins stacked up to our heads were sorted by age and sometimes gender, heaped with supplies, games, music, toys, and accessories that they could give to kids at hospitals when fulfilling wishes. I went to the Starlight office near Toronto more to fulfill a promise to Calvin than anything; another trail to follow to its conclusion, another opportunity to open up for my boy in case he needed it later.

The compassionate staff hadn't encountered gigantism before. No surprise, really. A couple hundred kids in the world and all. They promised privacy for Aaron and sensitivity for our family. A program director encouraged me to get Aaron thinking right away about what he'd wish for because it could take a little while to get things in motion, and Aaron would be nineteen soon, the maximum age of children the charity would fill wishes for. The wish needed to come from him, she reminded me.

I rushed to complete the paperwork. I was excited for Aaron. Something good was happening. I had no clue what he'd wish for. In fact, I'd been wondering in the dark hours if he still wished for anything except to turn the clock back, rid himself of the memories, and live in a world where people didn't stare. (And maybe for his hovering mother to vanish.) I told Aaron about my visit to Starlight, the application, and the warehouse of toys. I left the printed material for him in a pile on the ottoman where he did his homework.

"I don't need to see it, Mom."

"Can you think of something that you might want for a wish?"

"Nope."

"Will you try?"

"I'll try, but I really don't have any wishes. Not like little kids do. It's not like I ever wanted to go to Disneyland or to meet some famous player or a band or anything. I'd be embarrassed."

"You could ask to go to the Super Bowl," I nudged. He was a huge football fan.

"No."

I switched to baseball. "How 'bout Florida for Blue Jays' spring training?"

"No," he said. "I don't want anything like that. Forget it. I don't want anything."

I was a little upset. But I was making it about me. He was reacting like a teenager. I got that he didn't want to be embarrassed by meeting some famous player at centre field and posing for an autograph. Not his style. Aaron liked to be on the sidelines, knowing the plays, the coaching staff, and the player's profiles.

"I won't change my mind, Mom. Just tell them no thanks and they can help some little kid who wants to meet Mickey Mouse."

I said there were other children who would give anything to have their greatest wish granted.

"Then give the wish to another kid," he said.

"You'll lose your chance after your nineteenth birthday," Rick said.

"So what? I don't want it anyway."

Many times in the past, Aaron resisted but would later relent. Rick and I decided to let the application stand but I was honest with the organization that he might just say no. So I dropped it with him. I huffed away. We didn't speak about it for weeks. I told the Starlight volunteer we were concerned that Aaron would simply give up the opportunity to have a wish granted because he could not be bothered to come up with ideas. She reiterated the charity's priority that the wish come from the child and her discomfort in making any suggestions.

Aaron was in charge of this one and he was a tough customer. It had always been virtually impossible to change Aaron's mind when he dug in. We had a string of memories of restaurant dinners that ended in the parking lot, movies where we didn't get past the preview, and visits to places like Canada's Wonderland or the East Coast that had not happened because Aaron put a stop to it.

However, he agreed to sit down in a meeting with Michele, his bright-spirited personal wish-granter. For all we knew it might work better if someone official was encouraging him. For all we knew he might be as rude and negative about the whole thing as he was becoming with us. When Michele came over one evening, she brought hockey-themed gifts to the boys and talked to Aaron about different types of wishes, such as long-distance excursions or one-time events, like going to a concert. She mentioned a couple of unique wishes that other teens had been granted, trying to prime Aaron. I bolted my mouth shut. I neither egged him on nor ended the meeting before he had plenty of time to digest all the information. Resistance remained.

He even said no to the offer to join the Starlight private box at the Air Canada Centre, home of Aaron's beloved Toronto Maple Leafs, something that was available to Starlight wish kids on a regular basis. He refused many times. Aaron said he wasn't interested. I was shocked. And miffed and embarrassed to be turning down the Starlight generosity repeatedly. "Okay, Aaron, what's the deal?" I asked. "Why do you not wanna take anything you're offered?"

"I feel stupid, Mom." I wondered if stupid really meant scared.

"But it isn't like we're gonna drop you off alone to hang out with adults in suits or strangers or something … We would all be there. Do it for your brother, if you don't want it for you," I lobbed in at last and then prepared to be blasted.

"I guess it wouldn't suck too bad then."

Teenagers.

All four of us donned our Leaf jerseys and went two nights later.

The private box had different food stations, like concessions, serving kid-friendly food placed around a large room above a forty-person seating area with an incredible view of the ice. Aaron and Justin were into the hot dogs and fries and snacks right away, watching as other families arrived and shouting out answers as pre-game trivia went by on the huge four-sided screen suspended from the arena's roof. The boys leaned over to Rick or me many times to whisper how cute some nearby little person was. There were toddlers and school-aged children dressed in Leaf jerseys and toques or Starlight T-shirts, and others had shirts with messages, like *My brother is a cancer survivor.* Before we knew it, our two enormous boys were on their hands and knees carrying one and sometimes two children around on their backs. They were holding the hands of little ones who could not reach the pizza and passing food to others who could not leave their wheelchairs to get snacks. Rick and I beamed and left the boys to savour being needed and adored, stepping back together, just smiling. It was always so hard to get Aaron to try things, but it was pure joy when he liked it. His introversion was exactly like mine. I should have gotten this. *Duh.*

Aaron waved and played peek-a-boo with a little boy seated near us, who was obviously very sick, given his bluish pallor, dependency on feeding tubes, and limp limbs. The little boy smiled at Aaron, loving the attention from a big guy.

"See Mom, this is who the wishes are for."

"Littler kids, you mean?" I asked.

"No, the sick ones. This stuff should be for sick kids."

He doesn't think he's one of them.

"You have a lot in common with these kids, buddy."

"But I'm not sick."

"Yes, you are." He stole a glance at my face, maybe checking to see if I was crying. "You have a lot in common with these kids, Aaron."

Then we were both silent.

A couple months later, after polite check-in emails and urgings from Michele, I asked Rick to try one more time to sit down with Aaron and consider even small things he might need, rather than elaborate things he might want. I couldn't consume the charity's time any longer when it looked like Aaron wanted nothing at all. Rick suggested things that were Aaron's size. How about a computer with a keyboard with larger keys? Mentioning needs over wants got the list flowing.

"I need a bigger bed," he said to Rick, joking.

Fact was, there were a lot of things Aaron needed because of his size. He slept in the fetal position or corner-to-corner on a queen-sized bed. It was very difficult to get pants long enough, running shoes large enough, or hats in his size.

One day Aaron came bursting into the house and yelled, "Mom, I thought of something. Something I can ask for that I can live with getting."

Sports equipment. He wanted to be able to stay active and hoped it would help him stay pain free. "I could ask for golf clubs my size and skates my size. Then I would have a winter and summer option."

Custom-fitted Callaway clubs and all the accessories arrived a couple of months later. In the fall Aaron and I went to the Starlight offices to pick up right-sized skates, shoulder and shin pads, and best of all, a hockey stick (a copy of the one used by Zdeno Chára, the tallest player in the NHL) that fit Aaron, who was then six foot ten.

All this talk about wishing had me musing over my own so-called bucket list. And I realized, I didn't have one. I'd righted myself after the worst of the depression, managing now to consider my writing again. But I didn't dare to dream further ahead or more lavishly than what I was going to do for work. Former wishes, those I'd had the courage to consider when I faced being single, were all unachievable now. Once I would have wished for, and in fact planned on, a doctoral degree. And I wanted to live in Ireland — not exactly a trip to Hawaii — a bit more adventurous, but seriously, it was Ireland not Botswana. And I wanted to know an elephant. I never thought my bucket list would be reduced to a solitary item when I was forty-five years old: Let my children live a long and healthy life.

We had no way of knowing what would come next. We sat on chairs (far too small for Aaron) in a hallway where donors' names were more prominent than the signage announcing functions of the clinics, offices, and exam rooms. We were there for Aaron's appointment with the neurosurgeon Dr. Ezzat had referred us to. This was about next steps for Aaron, which could include surgery or radiation, or both, or neither. Because his numbers were still rising.

New hospital, new routine. It was uncomfortable to be in an unfamiliar space, a reminder that he was facing another round of treatment. I didn't like not knowing what to expect that day. I'd not been able to prepare him, answer questions, or anticipate decisions that might have to be made. The medical system wielded its mighty sword far too often in our lives and I resented it. We might be told that Aaron would be scheduled for sixty days of treatment. We'd been told that fractionated radiation for a pituitary tumour would involve daily treatments on weekdays over two months. That would mean an entire summer of commuting, a total of three hours each day for us. Another option was the single treatment called Gamma Knife, a type of radiation that was delivered through beams at multiple angles. And for all I knew, it could be booked that afternoon.

On days like that we hoped for pleasant interactions to ease our nerves, break up the ruminating, and give us anything else to focus on. But sometimes the office assistant wouldn't even look up from the desk when she took Aaron's card and checked him in. "Her loss," we'd mumble to one another as we sat down. She'd missed out on the Frick and Frack Show, on Aaron's gloriously *giant* smile ("Good one, Mom"), and the joy our goofiness would have brought to her day. We weren't being generous, and it certainly wasn't extroversion — we yucked it up because we needed to, and maybe also because we truly found ourselves hilarious. (I wondered if that was the final sign that we were totally losing our shit.) It wasn't intellectual humour and it wasn't gallows humour, it was our own adaptation of slapstick. It was the coping skill I pointed to when people asked, "How the hell do you stay sane?" It kept us normal. It kept us together. We were living in the theatre of the absurd, and teenage-boy humour grounded us like punks on the bus, removing our titles of mother and son, and gelling us as buddies in bad times.

"That never gets old," Aaron said, after having his blood pressure, weight, and height taken at registration.

"What doesn't?" I asked, walking straight into his joke.

"Watchin' the intern's eyes pop out of their head when they see my blood pressure. It's like getting the high score after not playin' fair … They all do a double take to check the numbers but I really think that second look is to check if I'm a giraffe!" He slapped his own thigh, he liked that one so much.

"Because your numbers are so *high*, ya mean?" (See what I did there!)

"They act like they've never seen anything like it! Come on, Mom. My numbers are nearly in the two hundreds. I should get a fuckin' medal for that!"

"I'd give ya a medal," I piped in. "A *giant* medal."

"Not bad, lady, but you've had better."

We sat in the quiet a while, checking the time on our phones every few minutes. Another forty minutes passed, and still we sat. He was getting hangry and I wanted more coffee but we couldn't leave, because we would lose our spot or get rescheduled, and that would neither assuage my anxiety about getting him cared for as quickly as possible nor guarantee that Aaron would be agreeable about coming back.

"Do you think they forgot us?" he asked.

"No, buddy, they didn't."

"Right, we checked in. Somewhere ten strangers are standin' over my file askin' each other what crap news they can unload on us to fuck with my life today. And we sit here helpless. I freaking love this." He'd come by his sarcasm honestly. I had no words, because I shared the sentiment and the attitude, on steroids.

When Aaron's name was called, we followed the reception staff into a dimly lit meeting room where about twenty white coats sat around a square table, their faces turned to look at a massive projector screen hung on one wall showing an MRI. *Maybe they do an intake round at this hospital,* I thought. *But this is serious overkill for an intake.* A slim woman with skin like butter and a dark sleek ponytail stood as we entered and invited us with a hand gesture to take the two empty seats. The conversation hushed to silence as we noisily sat. Aaron couldn't fit his legs under the table so he turned sideways, facing my profile.

"That's fine, buddy, just be comfortable," I said, tapping his knee as I scooched my chair over, making room for his legs. Then I got my first look at the faces around the table. Some were craning around those in front, trying to get a look at us, or rather, at my boy. The subject. The patient. The giant.

Dr. Maddow, Dr. Gentili's neurosurgery second-in-command, began by asking a few questions — to the meeting room, not to us. Ironically, Aaron was not Gulliver to the Lilliputians, he was much smaller than them, one-twelfth their size. We had deflated, lost our human-ness, our right to be treated as persons. Aaron's disease was the main character in this meeting, and my boy was only the skin covering it.

Dr. Maddow opened the room to questions, and I sat in the silence, my anger full in my chest. Like a helium balloon, I'd puffed up, shifted a little to almost be in front of Aaron, my body now partially obscuring their view of him. Still they said nothing.

I nodded my head toward the screen. "Is that him?" I asked Dr. Maddow, who was directly across from me.

"Yes, that is your son's MRI."

I glanced at Aaron. His shoulders had rolled in. He was fidgeting with the threads on his jeans, his eyes on the floor. He was prey in the crosshairs, trying to avoid detection.

I took a breath, then said in a measured tone, "You mean to tell me that you have a child with gigantism in the room, undoubtedly one of only a couple you will ever see in your esteemed careers" — I cleared my throat (I would not cry today) — "and you don't even have a question for him, something to learn from him?"

Like a classroom of high-school English students who hadn't read their *Macbeth* pages, their heads collectively slanted down to their laps.

"We're done here, Aaron."

And with my boy in front of me, we left.

Before my second foot was across the threshold, Aaron said, "Wow, you nearly lost it, Mom. Like, even for you, you almost got rude. You kicked ass."

Firm, maybe. Tough at my worst. *Or is it best?*

I had one operating instruction: Do not resort to rudeness. This was not a stint in emerg where pushiness might get him seen faster. We were part of an electronically managed system where humans rule and things happen at a glacial pace. Even though I had no idea what the expected outcome of this meeting was (until much later), I'd figure it out. And in the meantime, my kid was not going to participate in their freak show. Not on my watch.

The receptionist called after us, extending a piece of paper. "Your next appointment." I folded the page without looking at it and slid it into the fat turquoise medical binder.

20

MOTHER OF MEGATRON

"No, Mom, really. You should totally come with me."

This kid could talk me into anything. He sat with his legs stretched across the room, barring my walking by. "You should come to school with me on my short day. You could write while I'm in class and then buy me lunch after," he said, with that huge grin plastered on his face.

"It's all about the free food, isn't it?"

Another of our standing jokes. But now that he was commuting to the university and paying some of his own way, Mom's contribution was even more welcome than usual.

"Totally!" he said.

"Charming," I responded.

So I went with him one day. I knew he'd think moving my speed was a total pain, but he wanted me around and I wasn't going to refuse that. They'd be sick of me soon enough. On the commute he boasted about how he had it all memorized now, the way from our home into the Toronto downtown core. He knew where traffic backed up and which lane the bus needed to be in to not get slowed down. He had moved so quickly from a boy learning to drive, backing my SUV into a stanchion in the parking lot, to the independent and self-assured city student.

I loved tromping along, backpacks on, almost being carried by the stream of commuters. It reminded me of my own days as a student. I felt nostalgia with a side of longing for a life change (and wanting to be cool, so he wouldn't regret me coming along). Even if I'd been in good shape (and I surely wasn't) I couldn't have kept up with Aaron's fast-paced, super-long strides. I felt like the Merrie Melodies skit of the dogs, Chester and Spike. I couldn't stop looking at him. Partly because seeing him up ahead (and up above) was how I didn't get too far behind but also because I kept looking where everyone else was looking. And everyone was staring at my son, and most people didn't have the sensitivity to be discreet about it.

I saw him there in the crowd as different than me, than them. It made me ashamed, but as soon as I felt sympathy for him and peered up into his face (which prompted him to look down at me), he beamed his bright smile. We said nothing. *Did he just catch me glimpsing what it was like to be him?* Maybe he was smiling because I just saw that he didn't give a shit about what people thought of him anymore. He felt the stares, but he just went on about his business, swimming in his lane, living in his silo. I was so proud.

And he was adorable! We both stood under the handrails that are suspended from the train-car ceiling, and my arm was fully extended to grasp the rail, elbow locked open. Aaron was resting his forehead on the bar. I don't know why it struck me as cute. But it did. He was different. He knew it. He was mine. Better still, I was his. And in the wordless way we had learned to live for years in the After, we went to school.

Two pieces of news shifted the landscape for us after Aaron's first year of university. First, Justin's blood work showed no sign of inappropriate endocrine values, and the relief was immense but came with a caveat that I was already critically aware of — the disease could show up at any time, in any of us. (To this day, I watch him far too closely and make him crazy with questions about changes in his face, hand, and foot size.)

And second, Marta Korbonits's team in the UK reported that Aaron's gigantism could not be explained by the AIP genetic anomaly. As far as the study found, we were not related to Charles Byrne. I took this as good news but realized that this didn't place us any further ahead when it came to guessing Aaron's prognosis. There wasn't time to project, because Aaron's radiation treatment needed my full attention.

We timed the Gamma Knife radiation so that Aaron would be done his school year and still be able to have a summer job. We were told to expect no recovery time. It was a one-shot deal, and we were thrilled that Aaron would have one day of therapy instead of sixty. It would also mean avoiding the potential side effects of traditional radiation. But nothing could have prepared us for that day.

Aaron had gone in alone so they could prep him for the radiation treatment while we sat in small waiting room out of the main area. When I came around the nurses' station to find him, I think my heart stopped; my feet may have as well. He was sitting in a chair beside his narrow gurney, wearing two blue hospital gowns that barely went to his knees — one on frontward and the other backward, and neither was his size. Then again, few clothes are. I briefly scolded myself for not insisting that they let him wear his sweatpants. He deserved more dignity. Yes, even more than other people, if my inner truth be told. He was still a kid, if nineteen. I looked down to his feet — anything to avoid looking at his face yet or his head or the huge metal frame that was attached to it. There were the black leather high-tops. A hospital gown and Nikes. What an outfit!

Then my eyes locked with his. What was that? Terror? I couldn't name it. Glassy-eyed or was it teary? Or perhaps I saw pain. It felt like he was reeling me in; my pace quickened the last twenty feet or so. I dumped my books, purse, and his bag of belongings on the floor and crouched in front of him, my hands on either armrest of the chair he was squeezed into.

He needed to speak first. *Talk to me, son. Talk to me.*

Like his mouth was full of marbles, tears popped off of his lips as he spoke. "I hate this, Mom. I don't care if this might cure me. This is way worse than surgery. I haven't even done the radiation yet and I know I'm never doing this again. I nearly passed out when they were putting screws into my head. Screws in my fuckin' head. Why the hell wouldn't they put a person to sleep for this?"

Helpless, I looked over my shoulder to a nurse, asking if he could have a blanket. One arrived.

"They did it right here," he said.

"Where, here?" I asked.

"In this chair, in this huge open room. With a drill. A fucking drill, Mom. I started to sweat and they put a stupid fan on me."

"Your blood pressure must have spiked."

"I guess."

"Did the fan help?"

"I cried, Mom. They wiped some cream on me where the screws went in but it did nothing."

I had no idea why he wouldn't have been made more comfortable. Perhaps full lucidity was required during radiation. Or perhaps humanity is forgotten when doctors and technicians are more amazed by the use of radiation than they are concerned with the person under the titanium frame.

Aaron's tears had started again, but miraculously, mine were holding at bay. He went to wipe his eyes but bumped into the frame, which went entirely around his head at eye height, and winced. I took a tissue and reached under the bar to dab at his eyes. This upset him even more and the tears came for both of us.

There were four sites where what looked like flat-ended pins went through the square frame and pressed into his flesh — two on his forehead and two behind his ears, lost entirely in his hair. There must have been quite a bit of blood. Attempts to blot it had left smears around the bases of short metal posts. Where the pins touched, the skin was already inflamed and raw but not bleeding right now anyway. We'd learned in an information video that the head frame was to hold him still while a plastic helmet was placed over the frame with markings on it to guide the radiation specialists to locations on his head.

Barbaric bullshit. *Someone just put four screws into my son's head. And I let them.* I stood outside while they did it, and sipped coffee, wished I was dead or at least in the chair instead of him, while some overeducated, likely famous brain surgeon screwed titanium into my boy's skull. While three others held him down, he would tell me later. This may as well be a torture chamber. Glancing around me, I saw beds, curtains, wall connections for oxygen, but no other signs of torture, per se. This was enough. Loving mothers did not stand outside and wait, or use self-distancing phrases: "We have to do this" and "It's going to help you, *maybe* in a couple of years."

And then it was time. The nurse turned the oversized burgundy wheelchair away from me. I saw the metal bars protruding from the back of Aaron's head. I thought I'd throw up.

Self-loathing does not cover how I hated myself that day. But he was the one who had to go through it. As he rolled away, his head of almost-black hair beneath the scaffold-like apparatus comforted me, because I knew that head, my child, that fortress of a boy. My feet felt glued to the floor and I resisted my instinct to run after him, hug him, and push his horrified embarrassment to the maximum by telling him I loved him and could not bear the thought of living without him. My building panic was stopped by the hand of his brother on my back. I looked over my shoulder to see the same dark eyes, vacant of emotion, solid, waiting to read what my face told him I needed. Justin just hugged me and I wailed into my boy's shoulder. Rick stood a couple of feet away. We'd been separated for nearly three years at that point, and reminding me of the days when the four of us hugged in a ham-and-cheese-sandwich, he put his arms around both of us, and we bobbed like a cork in the sea of our memories.

The day before, I'd been anxious, unable to focus, my emotions so heightened that every worry bore equal weight — my disorganized closet, a light left on all night, being out of milk. Each of these was on the worry docket along with my son having radiation. Everything seemed important and yet nothing was, creating a mountain of problems I could not see over. So I started tearing everything out of my closet. The kids knew I moved furniture when I was happy and reorganized when I was worried. I had babbled something in reply when Justin had asked if I was okay. "Mom, you shouldn't have to do all this. You're exhausted."

"The closet?"

"Aaron," he said.

"You and your brother are my whole world, Jay."

"Dad can't handle something being wrong with one of us, can he?"

"No. Because he can't stand anything he can't fix." I left it at that.

Justin walked to me and just hugged me. It had been years since he just hugged me.

"My mom has too much to worry about," he said.

I thought of the description used by some of my friends who found themselves becoming caregivers and advocates to their aging parents ... that we become the parent in so many ways. Was that happening to Justin while I had my eyes on Aaron? Had Justin become the silent watchman, the protector of me? Was I in such bad shape or so perilously distracted that my son felt he had to care for me? I was not about to allow him to assume that responsibility, both because I was too tenacious and because it violated what I wanted for my kids: to just be them, not to be responsible for their parents' pain, mistakes, or failures. But I boxed up my concern for Justin and made a mental note to raise the topic with him when I had myself more together. He did not need to be my parent. I had to get my shit together so I didn't need one.

Every time they took Aaron, I relived every time before. Three years ago that very week, two surgeries through his nose took as much tumour off his pituitary as could be reached. Nineteen years before, a nurse carried my nine-week-old baby from me to attempt a risky hernia repair. I recorded these moments in my body, in my tissues, in the tense muscles of my shoulders, the stinging tear ducts. And while I waited for him to come back, I was without one arm.

Rick and I had fallen into a practised banter. We described imaginary (but quite possible) scenarios of how our usually good-natured, now gruff and surly, Aaron was likely bitching out the staff. We felt equal parts thankful we didn't have to be in there with him and sympathetic for the nurses who were. Justin said, "I must be the only kid who has divorced parents who have such a good time together. No one would believe it." In some effort to make himself such good company that he would always be invited to come on hospital days ever after, Justin was a one-boy comedy troupe that day. While Rick and I were gasping at the barbaric sight of a metal frame screwed into our boy's scalp and the crusted blood around the four points of entry, Justin nicknamed his brother Megatron and shouted, "Cool!" jumping up on the gurney beside Aaron and handing him a massive bag of chips. It was one of the few moments of lightheartedness in a horrific day. But it would be years before we would know if the procedure was successful at suppressing or shrinking the tumour.

In the following year, Aaron went to appointments with most of his doctors on his own. He would hike across the city from the university and handle his quarterly check-ins. But follow-up appointments with his neurosurgeon were something we decided to keep doing together.

One Wednesday afternoon appointment, just before the doctor entered the exam room, Aaron had been chattering as he does when he is nervous, going through what-if's and what the doctor might have to say after reviewing his latest blood work and MRI, which had just been done the day before. He was in the mood to rule out the worst-case scenarios. "Well, it isn't as if they'll do radiation again, 'cause the doctor said I could only have it once in my life, I think."

"Uh, no, that's not true. Radiation will be done again if it didn't do enough the first time."

"Well, I know for sure they won't operate again, 'cause Ezzat said surgery was the silver bullet — that they'll hold off until everything else has had a chance."

"Uh, no, that's not completely right either," I said, surprised by his presumptions. "Both radiation and surgery are options if the radiation didn't knock the tumour back. We know your IGF-1 is increasing and the radiation needs more time to do its thing." He pondered my responses. I was amazed that he had adjusted the information for himself to rule out procedures that doctors had indicated would be possible and even likely. It made me sad yet again to be the voice of reason, the bearer of doom.

Dr. Gentili came in, quickly shook Aaron's huge hand with his two more delicate ones and sat down in the chair facing us. The room was so small and the seating area so confined that we were almost touching one another knee to knee. I noticed Aaron rolling his chair slowly backward to gain some personal space. Nearly an hour and a half had passed since we'd registered, met interns, and repeated annoying, random details of Aaron's case history with that day's first-round physician. Aaron rocked his feet back and forth. I was on duty. I knew we had less than five minutes with the man who might one day operate on my son and who would lead the team to decide the next steps in radiation treatment, and we needed to learn everything we could and come away with a plan.

"How have you been feeling?" Dr. Gentili asked, looking at the page of notes he held on top of a manila folder in his lap.

"I'm good."

"That's it?" the doctor replied, chuckling a little.

Nothing from Aaron. I just smiled, hoping Aaron would take charge. Now I was the one being delusional.

"Well, the MRI looks good. Maybe a very teeny, teeny change that might be due to the radiation being successful." Conservative optimism.

Is it safe to hope? I knew this was why Aaron had adjusted his interpretation of the medical updates. He was more comfortable in delusion. He'd taught me this one particular hospital day when I sat in the cafeteria with my then sixteen-year-old and talked about his death.

"Do you know when I'm gonna die?" Aaron had asked, tearing into a slice of pizza. His tone was casual, nonchalant even.

"I know what the doctors say." Dread rose high in my throat. I had promised to always tell him the truth. I felt like I was choking as I waited for him to ask. He chewed. I gagged.

"As long as one of us does," he said and reached for his third slice. The imaginary Coast Guard called off the search and turned for port. Hell, a cutter wouldn't be nearly strong enough anyway. In that moment, I became the Daenerys Targaryen of the medical system, perhaps not the mother of dragons, but absolutely a Dragon Mother.

21

ORPHAN

At some point I realized I was no longer waking up thinking, "Aaron has a brain tumour." But perhaps just to torture myself or because overthinking is how I embrace the world or, even more likely, because I'm a writer, I wondered what that meant. Had I become blasé? Was I processing? Was I moving forward? Guilt swept in. Was it like the adage about being crazy — a word I never used — but everyone seems to know this one: If you think you are, you likely aren't. It wasn't like I could climb off this ride. If he couldn't, I would not.

Aaron told me, in one of our numerous car rides together, that he lived between the appointments, between our car trips, and between the days his nurse came to the house to give him his painful needles every three weeks. He told me that he wouldn't let the disease define him, and shutting his mind to it whenever he could was how he tried to do that. That strategy, his mindset, caused me to reflect on how much the disease had indeed defined me.

Gigantism's presence loomed large in our daily lives. Aaron needed a special seat on a plane, could not purchase clothing in regular stores, and needed links added to watchbands. But more serious considerations affected our lifestyle — regular visits by the nurse, time spent filling out government documents and filing tax returns to ensure financial help, and staying on top of prescription renewals.

In the summer of Aaron's radiation, a rare opportunity for my entire family to be together inspired us to have photos taken. There were lots of comments in the arranging emails. "Just in case this is the only time we are ever all together" (my sister); "while we are healthy" (my mother); "while I still have a waist" (me); "while I still have my hair" (my brother); "while we can still stand our parents" (all five of the kids). Just one year earlier I'd wrangled the boys into a photo shoot with me with the excuse that I was writing a book and needed candid but professional shots done. These remain my favourite photos ever. The boys wore T-shirts that we designed ourselves and flung me like a ragdoll between them. They did a set of pictures in hockey jerseys (Toronto, of course) and another in coordinated shirts and ball caps. We played and we posed for some great shots. Aaron stood straight while I dangled a measuring tape to the floor and Justin crouched to record the number. I climbed a step stool to get to Aaron's height and, in nine images shot in quick succession, he made faces as I leaned in and tried to kiss him. These are the priceless rewards of learning that lesson: One phone call can change everything and we must never assume our child will be the one who is the exception.

The same patient photographer worked with the ten of us that day in studio: my parents; my sister and her daughters, Laura and Michelle; my brother and his daughter, Hunter; and my boys and me. The undercurrent for the adults was a sense that my father's health was weakening. Before we began, I suggested that the photographer shoot Aaron seated so that he wasn't as self-conscious, but while in studio, Aaron said he was happy to stand, and all went quite well.

When the proofs arrived though, Aaron saw himself standing head and shoulders above my father and his uncle and said, "Oh my God, Mom, I'm fucking huge." In one photo of just the men, they all wore fantastic grins, each a squinty-eyed match for my father's, which warmed my heart. Aaron was resting his elbow on my father's shoulder. It was comical and sweet. But that isn't what Aaron saw.

"Mom," he said, "look at the size of my arm — it's bigger than Poppa's head." I looked where he was pointing, and he said in a whisper, "Am I really that big, Mom?"

"You are, my darling."

Not long after, the boys and I stood in my father's hospital room, and once again I felt the importance of getting a photo, the need for a memento. That was what was prompting me to rifle in my purse for my phone, fumbling around keys, loose bills, fountain pens, folded and disregarded medical forms, desperate to have a picture that I might never be able to capture again. *Damn it all, Patti, why the hell didn't you think of this and have the phone in your hand the whole time?*

The stakes were lofty as I stood, feet rooted to the sanitized linoleum floor, quivering like a dog accidentally left outside on a rainy night, watching as my teenage sons said their goodbyes to my dying father. I didn't know if we would see my father's sly little grin and his sparkling blue eyes again. I needed this picture and not just because I was unwilling to trust my depleted memory with the details. Moments were more sacred for me now and I knew this moment would be hallowed. Savouring and recording milestone moments in my boys' lives had elevated in significance. Those rendered unremarkable to others were chiselled to a fine point for me, their puffed-up poignancy capable of taking me down completely. I lived differently than I used to. I tasted the profound more than others. I had learned one truth that the happily oblivious rest of the world didn't know — life as if you know it can change in an instant.

In my father's hospital room, my mental camera pulled way back, panned a wide shot, and when the imaginary movie crane hoisted high, I saw me standing there, arms hugging myself, my enormous son leaning over the bed where Dad rested back on a stack of pillows, weakened by his failing heart but still the essence of the greatest man I had ever known. It would have been a beautiful scene if I could have remained a voyeur protected by distance from the personal disaster unfolding. But ceaseless alarm bells clanged in my head. I was going to lose them both. Now, tomorrow, or in the months to come, I was going to lose them both.

I pressed the button on my iPhone like a crazed paparazzo, expecting fully that tears and tension would produce either nothing in focus or nothing in the frame at all. I didn't care. I was not going to miss this, even if taking the photo meant I wasn't savouring the moment as I should. Aaron's long arms and dinner plate–sized hands wrapped completely around and under his grandfather's shoulders. I watched, lowering the phone, scanning for otherwise innocuous particulars, like how their profiles mirrored one another and the way my father's wizened hand patted Aaron's broad back feebly, causing the tubes and tape on his IV lines to flop in the air.

"I love you, Poppa," Aaron whispered.

"I love you too, A-man," my dad managed. Then in a whisper, he said, "G'night." His voice cracked and my heart with it.

I mentally counted the extra seconds they sustained that hug, each one a testament to what they both knew was coming, to the love they silently shared and the heartache they each wished they could spare each other. In the only decent photo of that hug, Aaron had stepped aside, head bowed, wiping tears roughly from his cheeks with the sleeves of his red hoodie.

It could be the last time I would see my son hug his Poppa. The last moment these two men I adored would be alive together.

They both clung to life, if on different timelines and in varying degrees of peril. But I would outlive them both. I would lose them both.

How can it be that I can do nothing about this? How can I just stand here and let my Dad die? Did I ask for every test? Did I talk to every doctor? Double check the medication? I had. But I could not save Dad. And Aaron was incurable. I could do nothing but be in the audience and scream silently at the universe, *"Please don't take my son too."*

I know that right after, Aaron walked around the bed to stand behind me. I caught a photo of Justin hugging my father seconds later. That picture shows my father enveloped in Justin's hug, his beautiful head of grey curls (once honey-blond) over Justin's arm. It was not the photo I was most desperate to have, but it was the sweetest photo I managed to take in my father's last days.

My father was my lighthouse, the one person who could always make me feel important. But even my Dad's ability to buoy me up was not enough in the years when my coping needs exceeded the reach of my family, my then husband and closest friends. I had been surviving by floundering from crisis to crisis, gasping for air in between.

Aaron and Justin stood on either side of me a moment later and we all smiled through our tears as my nieces joined in a group hug with their Poppa. I felt a mixture of comfort and surprise as Aaron stretched his big arm across my shoulders. I edged in closer to him and a giggle escaped me when my head tucked fully under my son's arm. I felt Justin place his hand lightly on my head and then he leaned in to whisper, "Let's go, Mom. Poppa will still be here in the morning," as if he knew something the rest of us didn't.

The months following my father's death were laden with the grey blanket of dulled sensations, tears lurking just below the surface of every french fry (my father's favourite), every glance into my sister's blue eyes (she looks so much like my dad), and every repeat of one of his sayings (the family calls them Floyd-isms.) But joy emerges, riding the backs of smiles and giggles that eventually become possible, seeping like water without effort or intention through the cracks in the heartbreak and sadness. The boys and I could always, and still do, bring my father back by telling stories about that time Poppa said this or the way that Poppa used to do that, and once again, laughter helped us heal.

My boys were hilarious, irreverent, and goofy, as teen boys should be. They would play YouTube videos of packs of puppies in the snow falling over themselves and one another, or show me embarrassing family photos from Facebook, slapping each other on the shoulder or arm. Funny cat videos were my second favourite, next to the dog-shaming photos, which struck so close to home for us. One showed a gorgeous golden retriever with a sign leaning up against his legs: "I got into the pantry and left potatoes hidden all over the house." We would laugh and remind each other we had to think to do this when one of our naughty goldens did something similar, which was inevitable.

I would often still be giggling to myself long after I watched them half-wrestling and body-checking, banging the door frame on their way out of my bedroom at night. The three of us always seemed to gather in a bedroom doorway or on the end of someone's bed after I'd abandoned the kitchen cleanup, and they their homework, or we were back from hockey practice, or the good television was over. It felt simple and normal, like everything hadn't been wrecked, like I told myself on the darkest days it had.

Once they left, I would sometimes journal for an hour — scrawling that became the skeleton of this book. I was always too stirred up to sleep. It was typical that around 11:00 p.m., because our rooms all opened into a common area with doors facing one another, a three-way conversation of shouts and jokes and stories would start. Often the two of them would end the night on the couch in my room or on my bed with our dogs.

These were sweet mommy moments for which I was most grateful; and they were the times when I was closest to tears. When the tears slipped out, the boys would gently tease me, using high-pitched, pseudo-Mommy voices: "Mommy likes having her little boys around." But the tears were a boiling over of a steadily percolating inner rage, if I was to tell the complete truth. These beautiful, joyful moments when we were all connected was when I was most tempted to spew at God, when I felt the most abandoned by a supposedly generous deity, and when I succumbed to the powerful sense of helplessness.

Aaron often had a story about the rudest thing that happened to him. "So, I'm on the subway and she comes right up to me and pokes her finger in my chest and says, 'How tall are you?' You wouldn't believe it, Mom. It was so funny, she had to reach up because she was probably a foot shorter than you, and I just looked at her. I should have said, 'Hey Lady, don't touch me' or something but I was so surprised. I just said, 'Boo!' Then she wandered away down the platform. And I thought the ones who mouth off at me are bad! This one was totally creepy. They're touching me now."

I realized things might be getting worse for him in the world. While some people knew that they should not approach, let alone touch a child, Aaron was now being treated like an adult, and the voyeurs were losing any sense of propriety.

But there was another change, one that delighted me. Aaron's confidence had bloomed during his years at university. He was new to Toronto and he enjoyed telling me that a place I used to visit in my university days had moved or was long since out of business. These updates reminded me that I was old, and if I didn't get that point, he was happy to tease me about my age. Sometimes he would tell us about a professor who was ridiculous or boring or beneath expectations. I was thrilled to see him live as if the spectre of the disease wasn't hovering over him.

Everyday conversations were pure bliss for us. When Justin described something he was pissed off about at school, he would wonder aloud whether Aaron had to do that too. The boys could talk about anything, and I was always so pleased to let them banter on because I knew another quiet time of intense stress and worry would take the calm from us.

But there were challenges being in our stressed-out family. The boys still stayed home a lot more than other kids their age. One day after school Justin mentioned that the guys on his hockey team were asking him why he never went drinking with them. They were all legally under age but the partying had begun anyway.

"Are they making it tough for you at hockey?" I asked.

He hesitated, looking from Aaron to me, and shrugged his shoulders. "Not really." He was lying. His confidence wouldn't let him admit it to me or in front of Aaron. But we all knew.

Rick and I talked often about how the boys were doing. We spoke about the fact that neither one seemed to want to be part of the parties with their friends and hockey teammates. We agreed to encourage them to go out, saying over and over that we wanted them to have as normal a life as possible, especially after our separation. The result of our encouragement though, was the boys' vehemently telling us they didn't want to party like their friends, and they were firm about it.

"You know, I want you guys to go out," I told Justin one day. "I'm totally happy being here writing on my own. Don't stay here because you think I need looking after."

"We don't, Mom, seriously. It's our choice, both of our choices, to not wreck our lives. You should be happy about it. Be proud of your incredibly fantastic kids," he said playfully. I didn't raise it again.

I know that it had been a social challenge for Justin to be the little brother. When Aaron returned to school in Grade 11, Justin had entered Grade 9, and everything that one of them did got back to the other. Aaron and his friends would tease and cajole Justin, calling him Guppy because he was the little fish in the figuratively large pond of high school. Justin couldn't do anything, from skipping class to eating ice cream at lunch, without Aaron knowing. And in most cases, without Aaron telling me, and that led to some very typical sibling tension, which I secretly celebrated.

One night, when Justin left our late-night chit-chat session, Aaron stayed sitting on the couch in my room. He was on his knees, with his elbows and forearms supporting him while he half lay on the couch to pet Reef, who was asleep on the cushion.

"I saw this sign today," he said.

"Oh yeah?"

"It read, *I'm going to live forever — it's going pretty well so far.* I thought that was a pretty cool one."

"Yeah, it is."

"I can say the same thing," he said, running his hand along the back of Reef's neck. "Except I make up my own version. *I'm going to live forever, my own forever.* It's true, after all."

I smiled and nodded, pinched back tears and sucked in my lower lip. Aaron wasn't looking at me. He was sharing a piece of agony, which had been silently weighing on him, for how long I couldn't know. I'd wanted to believe that he hadn't been paying attention. *He really knows.*

I had nothing to offer him but my nodding. I must have looked like a pyjama-clad bobble-head doll.

I waited for more. This conversation had to be his choice. I was not about to urge him on or shut him down by placating him.

He ran his massive hand down his dog's back, and a couple of minutes later, buried his face in Reef's neck. The truth of his prognosis, to whatever degree he understood or surmised it, hung between us like a dry-ice sheet, neither of us willing to confirm or deny its existence and both of us hating its presence.

I'd long wondered if he had any sense of the worst prognosis. My girlfriend Val asked me if I thought he knew and I blew her off. No way. If he knew, he would tell me, I felt certain. He would question me, ask me to get him better doctors, wouldn't he? Or was it possible he didn't tell me what he knew because he was protecting me. Who was the caregiver here?

I felt no relief in his possibly knowing the worst of the medical information I carried around with me. I felt pained that my boy should have to contemplate his life's end at a time when most kids would be feeling and acting invincible. I had been inflicting the truth on him from the beginning, albeit only as he demanded it, but it was me acting on him. As pleased as I was to think he was understanding and processing it somehow, my stomach turned. If he accepted it and even got to the point where he could speak openly about his shortened lifespan, then I faced the greatest fear — that one day I would be without him. His denial could no longer be my subterfuge.

22

STORY KEEPER

Val and I still wonder exactly how we found our way back to one another. Like a bird with one of its wings injured, we spiralled without one another. Balance brought us back together. Balance and need. She took a trip to the West Coast, and finding herself on the verge of a life epiphany, reached out to me by text. We just kept talking. We didn't rehash the mental or emotional condition I'd been in, how she had supported me and I'd rejected her, or what we'd not done to protect our friendship. We just stepped back into one another's lives. We'd lost enough time.

"Don't throw those out," I bellowed at Val when she waved two folded pieces of bristol board over an open black garbage bag. We were purging my basement for a downsizing move. She held one red and one white piece of bristol, each folded in three for the Grade 10 Careers triptych assignment, which Aaron and Justin had each done in high school. They were worn on the seams and dirtied, with pictures from magazines flapping where the glue no longer held.

"Those are my kids' dreams."

Aaron's was the project he'd been working on in the early weeks following diagnosis, the night before we met the doctors at SickKids, the night he got so upset at what felt like a futile effort to plan his future. He was still a long way from those dreams, but he had achieved so much. And he had time. Treatment had given him time.

A few weeks later, Aaron proudly walked across the convocation podium, and Rick and I let the tears drip off our chins just as we had when he graduated high school. It felt somehow like his achievements were bigger than those of other twenty-somethings. His sense of entitlement was more palatable. We snickered to ourselves that we were the only parents not having any trouble getting pictures of our kid.

"Sucks to have short kids," Rick said, grinning, to me, wiping his tears. Aaron wore a custom-length gown and the largest-sized mortarboard. We would have paid thousands for him to dress like his classmates and graduate at the university where both my sister, Kelly, and Rick himself (and two years later Justin as well) walked the stage to shake the chancellor's hand. He had survived surgery, finished high school and drug treatments and radiation. He did all that. And now he was receiving his bachelor's degree. It might have turned out so differently. Under the robe, he was the guy in the tailored navy suit, bought from a special clothing store. I was wrapped in gratitude, not avoiding remembering what we'd been through to make this milestone possible for him and knowing I would have done nothing differently, despite the heavy costs I was starting to realize I'd paid to my life, health, and happiness.

Not long after Aaron landed his "big boy" job in corporate-insurance claims, he happened to be car shopping at the same time that my lease was up and I was considering a new car.

"I'm looking at the new Civic hatchback," I said to him one night.

"Hey, so am I, let's go together and get a matched set!"

Tucked into the back seat of the sporty little car while I test drove, Aaron talked incessantly, problem solving all the issues he might have with the car. He was so excited to be buying a brand-new car with his own first few saved paycheques. I wanted the car because I figured it was the last time in my life I could go sporty and be impractical, and it was sweet. He wanted it because it looked "hot." When it was his turn to test drive, his head rubbed on the headliner of the car's sunroof.

"It's fun, but I'm not gonna fit," he said. He stopped the car and walked away. He'd figured out a contortionist's method of getting into little cars before and was used to stretching his right leg all the way to the gas pedal while sliding into the seat and under the raised steering wheel as he brought his knee up the side of the steering column. His knees would be nearly at the top of the steering wheel. It looked like he was driving a go-cart. I bought the Civic, and instead of feeling the sting that his size limited his choices, he turned his attention to an SUV and bought it. Cash.

He was also handling more things medically. I still received email notifications when his blood-test results were posted, and occasionally I would send this information to Dr. Korbonits in England (and once I met in her in person to discuss Aaron's case because she was interested in following his progress). After one appointment, Aaron texted me that he'd been prescribed some drug he'd never heard of and he didn't know why. I translated this into, "Mom, is something going on?"

Just as mothers forget the pain of labour until the horror is reactivated at their second birthing session, I felt as though I was a retired droid jolted back into its repetitive activity. In seconds, I was on the computer searching drug names, indications, dosages, and diagnostic variables. The haze of possible outcomes, MRI results, and symptoms flooded my mind in a way that I'd been immune to for a few years. I was on duty again, my grown son's Grizzly Mom.

Aaron was mildly bothered. He didn't want to be recalled to the downtown hospital for frequent blood work that would be required to begin the new drug regime. He was annoyed. I was terrified. There we were at the crossroads of our present and our past, each responsible for how we'd managed during the scariest years and both wondering how the roles might work if a new health crisis was upon us. I was sucked into the medical TARDIS, back to the skills and the fiercely curious posture I'd adopted before. And deep within me the low rumble of the fear mantra was on repeat: *Please, not my baby … Please, not my baby …*

It all came rushing back. The blurred years of depression, the career goals I'd long since packed away, the choices I'd made, and I saw only the quiet, lonely, compartmentalized life I'd settled for. I felt like one of those Boxing Day shoppers careening maniacally through crowded aisles of electronics, shoving stacks of boxes, people, and carts out of my way. I needed answers NOW! It was bigger than me; it was all the love I'd ever known poured into whatever actions I could muster to ascertain what had caused Aaron's clinical team to prescribe a drug we did not know he needed. I birthed a crisis that was mine because it was his. I logged into the hospital medical portal and line by line combed the pages of clinical notes and more than thirty blood results. I learned that Aaron's growth-hormone levels were no longer responding to treatment. His graph line was climbing. He hadn't felt the symptoms yet, but his proactive endocrine team implemented an aggressive drug combination with the hope that it might have results before Aaron felt the disease's effects.

And it worked. Two months later, Aaron's levels were the lowest they'd ever been. It was a small storm, one that reminded us of past hurricanes and put us on notice that the chance of rogue waves was constant and permanent. Aaron and I always shared the tendency to overprepare, to anticipate worst-case scenarios, bracing ourselves for terrible news, hoping to be surprised by something less horrid.

"I guess I'm like this because I never had control over all the bad shit that happened to me," he said one evening, downing a third cup of *concoction* — the hot chocolate, French-vanilla cappuccino mix I kept simmering on the stove on the cookie-baking nights the boys still insisted on. "So I try to control things too much and it blows up," he said. "No wonder people think I'm a hard-ass."

He'd recently had his heart broken by a girl. "Why are you the only person who really knows me, Mom?" he'd asked. I wished he wouldn't hurt, as every mother must. But after I listened to him and gave him what balanced view I could on the events that led to his break up, I headed to my office and savoured this day deeply. It was all so *normal.*

It was a small sky-blue piece of paper.

Aaron was handing it down to me, where I sat, laptop poised on my knees, my booted feet surrounded by the cacophony of things I sherpa around on hospital days, a work bag stuffed with notebooks and manuscript pages for a couple of projects, a large carryall with my phone spilling out, my water bottle — because I never know how long we'll be. He wasn't waving it like the multi-starred test that would inevitably show his 100 percent in red Sharpie. He'd come up to me quietly, getting my attention because his body blocked the winter sun shining meekly through the atria skylight overhead. We're so bloody light starved in March.

I read his face. *Oh shit.* He was here to get me, not here because he was ready to go home.

The wail was fighting to become audible, tearing me open, just a low howl from deep inside. I could hear its vibration gathering muster, feel its power rising. It hadn't escaped from the darkness where mothers of sick kids bury their fear.

Please, not my baby ... And there it was, my sea-storm companion, the plea, the mantra, the prayer I'd devised ten years before.

What is his face saying? Had I stopped being able to read his pain, worry, despair? Had I gotten complacent because things hadn't gotten much worse for a year or so?

The gasp I made surprised people around me, what the kids and I called the Mommy Noise, that reactive air-suck of brake slams in the car and nearly spilled glasses of juice. I was still peering up at Aaron. He'd come back from the neurosurgery clinic after less than ten minutes. I'd settled into a lobby armchair to wait, leaving him to dodge signs and EXIT light boxes dangling from the ceiling on his way to the elevator up to the third floor because his MRI report from a couple of days before had been "unremarkable" — medical for nothing new and nothing worse, but nothing better either. But now here he stood. He needed me to come with him. The blue card was a test request, a note from his neurosurgeon, an appointment, I could now see, telling us where we needed to go in the hospital for the next thing, the next blade of steel in my son's side.

I took it from him. The three people sitting in the little four-chair cluster stared at me, willing me to hurry the hell up and tell them the news. You get used to living out loud in a hospital.

I righted it my way to read the handwriting in the pre-printed fields. My eye landed on the date. Like a beacon in the night.

2021.

That's two years from now. What? He comes here every few months ...

It dawned.

"Two years?" I said.

"Yup. I tried to talk him into eighteen months, but he doesn't need to see me for two years."

My eyes met those of the people seated in upholstered armchairs just a couple of feet away. They returned to their phones and books. Slow news day, we were. Nothing to see here folks …

Smoothies in hand — tradition on hospital days — we walked through the cold wind and a fledgling snow flurry to my car. He told me about his few minutes with his stylishly dressed older brain surgeon. "He didn't remember me, but I never expected him to …"

"Oh, come on. How many *yous* are there?"

I wasn't being a doting mom. Well yeah I was, but … what I meant was, how many patients does the man have that are almost seven feet tall and are being treated for a brain tumour?

"I don't know, Mom, maybe there are others and he can't keep us straight. Maybe he doesn't try. He's a brain surgeon, not a chiropractor."

The surgeon had asked whether he'd done Aaron's brain surgery and remarked on how it was almost the tenth anniversary of when he'd been diagnosed. "I told him he'd done my radiation seven years ago. He said, 'We think we're starting to see the radiation has had an effect. The tumour isn't active. You can be monitored closely by your other doctors.'"

Aaron stretched his arm over my head, splaying his hand at the top corner of the eight-foot glass door to the parking garage, holding it open for me. The same way he leaves his prints on my fridge door when he closes it.

"I wonder where we'll be in two years," he said. We sipped and walked. "I wonder *who* we'll be." I listened to the echoes of our two sets of footprints in the empty garage. Mine double timing his.

My boy was forward thinking, and not just a day, or to a time in the future beyond treatment, or to the next needle, *a couple of years*. But the musing ahead to calm seas didn't last, and he returned to heed the warning on the map in his mind. "Do you think I should have tried to get an appointment sooner?"

"I think if you're in trouble or the tumour is doing something, it'll show up in your blood. We'll have to make sure you get your blood work done every time you do the endocrine checkup. You always do, anyway, right?"

I watched him fold his legs into my car, his knees pressed up against the dashboard. The woman at the drive-thru coffee place earlier that morning had done a double (or a triple) take when she saw the size of the man in my passenger seat, which I had pretended to ignore. If we'd driven his SUV, he would've been much more comfortable. But he preferred I drive because I know the city so well, don't need a navigator, and don't mind the heavy traffic surrounded by aggressive, hurried city dwellers, but I suspected it was mostly because that's how we'd always done it.

"Maybe I won't still be living at home anymore when we come back," he joked. "I wonder where I'll be working?"

"We'll have to make a point of marking this day and flashing back to it when we come in two years," I said. "We should try and park in the same spot. This brand new garage that smells like fresh paint'll stink like the city by then!"

I ran a couple of scenarios about the two-year time frame in my head. What my life would be like. I was in a new relationship. Would it last? I was waiting to hear if my book had been picked up by a publisher. Would it be out? Would I still be so worried about money, still so afraid of ending up alone? Would I have gotten rid of the house I'm in, bailed on the housing market, finally made some decisions to say yes to opportunities? Would I have become brave enough to travel?

"Maybe you'll be living in California by then," Aaron mused. I had a client on the West Coast who had subtly suggested he would be supportive of me relocating. Aaron thought it was a cool idea.

"I don't know. It sounds amazing, but I'm a coward. I'm still working on dating. I'm an old lady afraid of her shadow."

I was edging into personal territory that I habitually spared Aaron and Justin from. We were close, but I didn't like to make my sons squirm nor did I ever allow them into my private life, such as it was.

He took the helm then. "Nothing has to be forever anymore, Mom."

"Whaddya mean?"

"Reef is gone now," he said. We had said goodbye to our beloved Reef — Aaron and I sobbing together, running our hands along the silky butterscotch fur and kissing the snout of the dog who had been our rock, our reason, our shared focus. I had never been more proud of the man he'd become, witnessing his gratitude for Reef's unwavering companionship at the same time repeating encouragement for me that I had always done everything right by that dog. We were alone in the agony, united by the shared loss that stretched thinly between our breaking hearts. "You've been the best friend I could ever've asked for," he told Reef, as the last few inches of tail managed a gentle wag.

"Reef is gone. I know the other pets still need you but your load is lightening. And I just got good news. Two things that have stopped you …" Aaron added, "I know you've been stopping yourself from doing things, feeling like you had to be here. Gooo, Mom." He made a shooing motion, his sausage fingers cantilevering out from his meaty hands, flick, flick. "Gooo. Ireland. California. Wherever. Write, hike, drink, whatever."

And then, the cherry on top, his punctuation mark, the reflection that a parent never wants to hear but knows is percolating within their children, "Don't you think Justin and I know that for the last ten years you've been living for *us*?"

Tears slipped down my face. I drove. He played with his phone. He doled out the wisdom and I inhaled the magnificence of the man he had been gifted the time to become.

He's still here. My every-morning mantra, the first thought of every day for ten years. Three thousand times I'd meditated on his survival, and now this. *He is coaxing me to live.*

"You can let go now. You let go of Reef. We can take care of everything here. We aren't assholes. We can keep your house standing and feed the cat. Gooo."

Could this be something he needs me to do? Had he been carrying the responsibility of feeling like he was the reason I wasn't striving for work away from our small town or adventuring to exotic travel destinations?

And then the intricacy of the past decade bloomed in front of me. In staying close, in keeping my life flexible in case he needed me, in living differently because his illness had exploded in our lives, had I made the pain of an altered life course more difficult for Aaron to bear?

I reached over and rested my hand on his arm. There would be waves, even storms, but he had the helm now, and I would need to become a trusting first mate.

Sail on, son.

A lot happened on the way to the epilogue.

EPILOGUE

MAPMAKER

Memoirs are maps, and the stories that compose them are the place markers. And as maps, memoirs require folding and unfolding, they get tucked away and yanked out, succumbing to crumpling in our rage and gentle compliance with our apologetic flattening out when we seek their wisdom in order to recognize our context. They are way-finding tools on harrowing journeys, and our companions as we travel home.

Before these pages there wasn't time or opportunity to analyze what happened to me; or maybe I hadn't been willing to turn my scrutiny from the waves long enough to gaze critically over my shoulder. I have concluded it to be the latter.

I naively believed we'd come up with a method for living with the spectre of Aaron's disease, something tangible, a way of being that included an awareness of how differently it might have all turned out. I faced the prospect of an epilogue with reticence because the ending — the one I sacrificed my marriage, friendships, career, and sanity for, the one that Aaron and to some extent Justin too truncated their childhoods for — did not come. Has not come, yet. I can't offer you a tidy ending, reader, no bow to tie up the pretty package. The destination we seek remains elusive for families like mine. Ours is a life in the unnamed geography after the After. Mine is not a book of miracles, but it is one of gratitude and celebration common to parents and family members who walk the halls of hospitals, do their work on laptops in waiting rooms, stay in touch with friends by text message from the bedside, and search Google into the wee hours after ensuring their loved ones have fallen asleep. We live in what Susan Sontag called "the kingdom of the sick" and there is no escaping the demands of its infrastructure. The comforting resolution at the end of a book does not come in the conventional form for *raremoms* and *warriordads*. Endurance prevails.

At the time of writing this, it is almost exactly ten years since the day I walked Aaron to his first brain scan. He has had a dozen MRIs since then. A small remnant of tumour remains, a fingerprint on the lens of the telescope through which he dreams his life. Perennial also is the treatment, the vigilance, and the reality that he cannot live with peace of mind or perhaps physical comfort without frequent visits to multiple doctors, that he must secure funding for his tumour-suppressant medication. Each sore muscle, strange skin pigmentation, headache, period of prolonged sleeplessness, or nose bleed could be *something*. There are also the bigger worries, the ones we still don't share with one another, like longevity, fatherhood, and his mobility, as if saying them out loud might fuel the likelihood of disaster, feed the monster that lays in wait. But we plod on, and our routines, our connections, and our giggles sustain us.

Sometimes Aaron walks into my kitchen while I'm chopping vegetables, and he starts in on a self-deprecating rant that is really difficult for me to hear. I want to tell him to stop, that he's wrong, that he's being too hard on himself, but we know each other too well. I can't play Mom to him. We've been cellmates too long. This is the child I coaxed into banking blood when he was terrified of needles, for whom I encouraged a second surgery that he might have refused if given full authority, when I knew there was a possibility he could die — and if he lived, might never forgive me for taking his autonomy away. We both share a penchant for blaming ourselves when the actions of others disappoint us. He gets agitated, self-judging, and *loud*, a floor-pacing beast trapped in a cage of his own creation. And it's like looking in the mirror.

Would we have been so much alike if fate hadn't thrown us overboard together?

I hear the door of Aaron's SUV slam in the driveway and smile as the dog skitters across the ceramic floor to press her wet nose to the window. Aaron always brings her Timbits; Tim Hortons must have had dogs in mind when it began selling the little donut holes. Aaron stops to tap on the glass and greet Tundra in the high-pitched training voice we were taught when Reef was a puppy. Aaron holds the red donut box up, just to excite her more. We're never sure if she wants the coffee more or the donuts, but Aaron shares them both with her. The tail wags, hitting the sides of the desk or a table leg like a base drum.

My heart skips a beat. Sometimes I even get butterflies. Aaron is home. *He is still here. He is still here.*

A LETTER FROM MY SON

This is not my story. That is to say, *Loving Large* is not my view of what happened or how I changed and evolved through my diagnosis, surgeries, and treatment. It is my mother's story, and one I think she should tell.

I have chosen not to define myself through this disease and the events of these years. This is just a part of me, and my viewpoint comes as much from me as it does from my mom, who helped get me through everything.

Without my mom, there is no way I could have made it through all of that.

I was sixteen. I was a scared kid who didn't understand what was happening while I was being treated. My mom took charge, did the research, understood the disease, the possible outcomes, and what was to come in the frightening time ahead.

Being diagnosed with a rare disease scared me but I did my best to bury the fear and the pain and act as if nothing was wrong. I was already one of the tallest kids at my school and did not want to be branded a freak. I wanted to be myself. I wanted to fit in, to exist in the background and not be noticed.

My mom encouraged me to be myself. She helped me not become depressed and made me feel like I wasn't alone. She became much more than my mom — she became my friend and the person I spent the most time with, not just because we went to multiple doctor appointments every week for months, but because she understood what was happening. She was part of it with me.

Things were not always good. We had extremely rough moments, and moments I'm not proud of. I felt powerless when the decision for me to have a second surgery was made, something I felt was very much out of my control and I lashed out at her. It bothers me to this day, years later — that I said what I said and did what I did to my mom, to the woman who was trying to save me.

As I said, this is not my story. This is my mom's story of her oldest son being diagnosed with a rare disease — one that I tried for so long to deny. I hid my pain for weeks and did my best to pretend nothing was wrong. In the end my mom saw the pain and fear. She helped me to understand what was going on without terrifying me with too much information or too many scary possibilities. She understood and understands the disease. And she carried the family through everything.

The cost of carrying both of us must have been enormous. If I didn't have her in my corner, I don't know what would have happened.

I look forward to supporting her, my mother the author, and this valuable book. Everyone finds our unique, fun-loving relationship infectious. I'm proud to share us with the world.

— Aaron H.

ACKNOWLEDGEMENTS

There should be so many people to thank. A memoir is a distillation of so many interactions, energetic connections, scenes, and experiences that rely on the existence of others. Since you've read the book now, you'll know that I chose to sail solo much of the time. But even a lone captain relies on her ballast.

My agent, Lisa Hagan, carried the proposal to Dundurn Press, where the team chose freelance editor Paula Chiarcos to wade through the marsh with me. It has been a pleasure to work with all of you.

My gratitude and much more extends to the medical experts who have come into our orbit in the last ten years. I cannot thank everyone, but I must mention personally the physicians who spent time with me in order to specifically contribute to this book, to my understanding, and to share in the wonder of gigantism. Dr. Michael Cusimano, Dr. Shereen Ezzat, Dr. Marta Korbonits, Dr. Cathryn Tobin, and endocrine nurse Lori Kingdon have each supported this work at one time or another through extended conversations, chats outside of clinic, or responsiveness to my queries.

Dr. Susan Kirsch (Aaron's favourite) kept in touch, emailed and met with me over ten years to relive the diagnostic months, savour Aaron's medical successes, remind me what we'd gone through, teach me what I could manage about endocrinology, and read through my pseudo-medical take on gigantism, as well as earlier drafts of *Loving Large*. The less-than-medical writing of medical elements is entirely my responsibility.

I'm indebted to the early readers of bits and pieces of what became *Loving Large*, the short list of memoir-loving, Patti-supporting writers includes Steph Jagger, Carly Butler Verheyen, Lara Heacock, Patricia Weltin, Sue Reynolds, CJ Schepers and Cate Emond, and members of the Beautiful Writer's Group, the web-child of Book Mama Linda Sivertsen, the manuscript's first unabashed fan. I kept a note Linda wrote me close at hand for the years it took to get this book baby to press, which read, "Patti Hall is a beautiful writer." She always believed it, even when I forgot it. Thank you, Linda, for everything you did for *Loving Large* in its nascent days.

My clients cheered from the sidelines as I proposaled, agented, sold, edited, and published, and they were sometimes more excited than I was: Dr. Mandy Lehto, Shelley Paxton, Giovanna Capozza, Teo Alfero, Gail Heald-Taylor, Deborah Bakti, Mary Louise Jarvis, Cheryl Wood, Gina Hatzis, and Allana Pratt. To the many others I've worked with in these years, I apologize in advance for not mentioning each of you by name.

The marvel that is the talented Maria Mutch was the first to read the completed manuscript. She has been my companion in memoir, Icelandic snowstorms, long writing deadlines, goofy animal voices, woodland wonders, mothering our sons, savouring beautiful things, and obsessing over coffee. She has been a compass.

My unwavering and brilliant coach, editor, and friend, Betsy Rapoport, chose to work with me and was willing to cry with me through all fifty revisions of the toughest parts while remaining sufficiently armoured to resist my anxious begging to hurry up and call the manuscript ready, already. You are the best thing that happened to my book and my writing life, Betsy. I never want to do this without you.

My nearest and dearest stayed tuned in to years of book updates and always managed to convince me they weren't bored yet with waiting for a real copy: Raelene, Colette, Erica, Michele, Vicki, and Ingrid.

My sisters in almost-DNA, suffering, and life choices, who know where the metaphorical bodies are buried and helped me do the digging, Miss A and Leni: You've fuelled me, urged me, reminded me, and scolded me for twenty-five and thirty-two years, respectively. You've seen it all. You've walked with me, sat by me, resisted my resistance, called me on my clever attempts at subterfuge, unconditionally believed and unabashedly cheered, and then loved me home. Thank the writing gods for both of you.

To "Rick," in your seat in the audience, thank you from the bottom of my grateful, fractured heart for having the single largest impact on my life and honouring me with the dudes.

My sun and stars (my sons and stars, as I call them) are my best work, the people I look up to (figuratively and literally), and their approval is enough, even though I realize I'll work the rest of my life wondering if I've earned it. I am so deeply proud to be Aaron and Justin's sidekick, their "Maaa!" Guys, please always choose me. I love you both so fiercely that it hurts.